Psychosomatic Medicine

Kurt Fritzsche • Susan H. McDaniel • Michael Wirsching
Editors

Psychosomatic Medicine

An International Primer for the Primary Care Setting

Springer

Editors
Kurt Fritzsche, MD
Psychosomatic Medicine and Psychotherapy
University Medical Center Freiburg
Freiburg
Baden-Württemberg
Germany

Michael Wirsching, MD
Psychosomatic Medicine and Psychotherapy
University Medical Center Freiburg
Freiburg
Baden-Württemberg
Germany

Susan H. McDaniel, PhD
Department of Family Medicine
University of Rochester
Rochester
New York
USA

ISBN 978-1-4614-1021-8 ISBN 978-1-4614-1022-5 (eBook)
DOI 10.1007/978-1-4614-1022-5
Springer New York Heidelberg Dordrecht London

Library of Congress Control Number: 2014933829

Printed on acid-free paper

Springer is part of Springer Science+Business Media (www.springer.com)

Preface

In 1978, representatives from 134 countries convened in Alma Ata, calling for "health care for all by the year 2000." (*Declaration of Alma-Ata*. 1978) This was a turning point for global mental health care, as this declaration emphasized the importance of health care near people's homes, health promotion and disease prevention services alongside curative medical service delivery, and mental health as an integral component of health. Thirty years later, Barbara Starfield elucidated the evidence to prove that countries with the best morbidity and mortality figures and overall health were linked to health care systems based on a strong foundation of primary care (Starfield et al. 2005).

In 2007, the *Lancet* published a series on global mental health, which identified the gaps in mental health care services, particularly in low and moderate income countries. Key works in this *Lancet* series (Movement for Global Mental Health 2007), followed by the movement for global health launched on the 2009 World Mental Health Day, provided the momentum and backing to work toward mental health care for all. (World Federation for Mental Health 2009). WHO and the World Federation for Mental Health have now joined forces to advocate for policies and practices to reduce stigma and integrate mental health into primary care systems.

In 2008, the World Health Organization (WHO) and the World Organization of Family Doctors (Wonca) published a report that delineates the need, describes best practices, and identifies 10 common principles for successful integration of mental health care into primary care. (WHO and Wonca 2008). This document, along with the works of Patel, Schirmer and colleagues provides tools, strategies, and best practices for mental health and behavioral health integration into primary care in low and moderate income countries. (Patel 2003; Schirmer and Montegut et al. 2010).

Since 2001, the Department of Psychosomatic Medicine and Psychotherapy of the University Medical Center, Freiburg, Germany, maintains exchanges with the Asian countries China, Vietnam, and Laos, with Iran, with African countries such as Sudan and Uganda, as well as with colleagues in other European countries and the USA and Australia. Ongoing classes in Psychosomatic Medicine and psychotherapy are held especially in Asian countries and Iran. In their feedback, hundreds of doctors, from young professionals to highly experienced doctors, reported to have benefitted tremendously from the courses both professionally and in their personal relationship with patients. The experiences we gained in these last 10 years with respect to the content, and pedagogical and methodological design of the courses are included in this book.

This book was written for curious doctors who wish to gain and develop knowledge and skills in Psychosomatic Medicine. The main question is therefore: How can I learn Psychosomatic Basic Care? Psychosomatic Medicine is a multidisciplinary subject involving extensive knowledge. It is not possible to treat all clinical manifestations in one class and in this textbook. Therefore, basic ways of thinking and approaches in the most common diseases are presented.

The book is organized according to the three objectives of basic psychosomatic care:

1. Recognizing psychological and psychosomatic conditions and disorders
2. Limited personal consulting and treatment services
3. If necessary, targeted referral to and cooperation with mental health specialists.

The book is divided into a general part and a part with specific clinical manifestations. The general part addresses topics that are relevant to all clinical manifestations such as the interaction between mind and body, doctor–patient relationship, doctor–patient communication, the family interview, and the Balint group. The second part addresses specific clinical manifestations that are most frequently encountered in primary care, including depressive disorders, anxiety disorders, somatoform disorders, posttraumatic stress disorder, alcohol dependency, and psychosomatics of life threatening diseases such as cancer and coronary heart disease.

Each chapter is divided into diagnostics, treatment, and pitfalls. In each chapter, typical case studies are used to demonstrate the diagnostic and therapeutic steps. As a result, the book has a high practical relevance, and can also be used directly as a course book in training in Psychosomatic Basic Care.

Kurt Fritzsche, MD
Michael Wirsching, MD
Susan H. McDaniel, PhD
and Julie Schirmer, BA, MSW

References

Declaration of Alma-Ata. International conference on primary health care, Alma-Ata USSR, 1978. http://www.who.int/hpr/NPH/docs/declaration_almaata.pdf. Accessed 22 June 2012.

Movement for Global Mental Health. *Lancet series* on global mental health. http://www.globalmentalhealth.org

Patel V. Where there is no psychiatrist: a mental health manual. London: Gaskell; 2003.

Schirmer JM, Montegut JA. Behavioral medicine in primary care: a global perspective. Oxford: Radcliffe Publishers; 2010.

Starfield B, Shu L, Macinko. Contribution of primary care to health systems and health. The Milbank Quarterly. 2005;83(3):457–502.

World Federation for Mental Health.World mental health day 2009: mental health in primary care: enhancing treatment and promoting mental health. World Federation for Mental Health; 2009. http://www.wfmh.com

World Health Organization (WHO) and the World Organization of Family Doctors (Wonca). Integrating mental health into primary care: a global perspective. Geneva, Switzerland: WHO; 2008.

Acknowledgements

We thank the more than one thousand medical colleagues who in the past 20 years have attended our courses and have provided us with valuable feedback to improve the content and didactics of the book. We want to encourage them to continue on their way to an integrated Psychosomatic Medicine. We thank Mrs. Sabine Rösler and Eva Schneid who have compiled each chapter patiently and painstakingly. We thank our administrative assistants Mrs. Kunz and Mrs. Engbers for completing the paperwork. We thank Mrs. Beth Schad of Springer for her support in the completion of the book.

For the sake of readability, in the present work collective terms (patients, doctors, etc.) are consistently used in the grammatically masculine form, however, both male and female subjects are encompassed equally.

Contents

Contributors

Catherine Abbo Department of Psychiatry, Makerere University College of Health Sciences and Mulago National Referral and Teaching Hospital, Kampala, Uganda

Hamid Afshar Zanjani Department of Psychiatry, Medical Faculty, Psychosomatic Research Center, Isfahan University of Medical Sciences, Noor Hospital, Isfahan, Iran

Frank Kuan-Yu Chen Division of Psychosomatic Medicine, Taipei City Psychiatric Center, Taipei City Hospital, Taipei, Taiwan

Gertrud Frahm Department of Human Sciences, Federal University of Paraná, Curitiba, PR, Brazil

Kurt Fritzsche Department of Psychosomatic Medicine and Psychotherapy, University Medical Center, Freiburg, Germany

Werner Geigges Rehaklinik Glotterbad, Glottertal, Germany

Farzad Goli Department of bioenergy economy, Energy Medicine University, California, USA

Danesh-e Tandorosti Institute, Isfahan, Iran

Wei Jing Department of Psychological Medicine, Peking Union Medical College Hospital, Beijing, China

Jeffrey F. Markuns Department of Family Medicine, Boston University, South Boston, MA, USA

Susan H. McDaniel Department of Psychiatry, Department of Family Medicine, University of Rochester Medical Center, Rochester, NY, USA

Sonia Diaz Monsalve Department of Psychosomatic Medicine and Psychotherapy, University Medical Center, Freiburg, Germany

Kim Viet Nguyen Department of Psychiatry, Hanoi Medical University, Hanoi, Vietnam

National Institute of Mental Health, Bach Mai Hospital, Hanoi, Vietnam

Van Tuan Nguyen Department of Psychiatry, Hanoi Medical University, Hanoi, Vietnam

National Institute of Mental Health, Bach Mai Hospital, Hanoi, Vietnam

Julie Schirmer Family Medicine Department Maine Medical Center, Family Medicine Center, Portland, ME, USA

Axel Schweickhardt Potenziale GmbH Business Consultants, Nuremberg, Germany

Michael Wirsching Department of Psychosomatic Medicine and Psychotherapy, University Medical Center, Freiburg, Germany

Lan Zhang Department of Psychiatry, West China Hospital, Chengdu, Sichuan, P.R. China

Xudong Zhao Department of Psychosomatic Medicine, Shanghai East Hospital Tongji University, Shanghai, China

Part I
Psychosomatic Medicine in Primary Care

Chapter 1
What is Psychosomatic Medicine?

Kurt Fritzsche

Case Study Initially, a 59-year-old female patient is hospitalized for removal of benign polyps. During hospitalization, in the context of thromboembolism in the right leg, a gangrene of the right toe develops. Other complications such as poor wound healing and infection lead to emergency amputation of the lower leg.

After surgery, the patient is alert and responsive, but appears to be desperate and helpless. After a few sentences, she begins to cry: Already when being transferred to the ward, she heard the nurses say that they were overwhelmed by her case. She feels pushed away, has little hope of improvement. She feels like "being a funnel into which one pours something on the top and everything comes out again from the bottom."

(to be continued)

Psychosomatic Medicine deals with the interactions between physical, emotional, and social processes in the occurrence, course, and the patient's coping with disease and states of suffering.

Example 1: "Asthma Bronchial" Psychosocial factors may co-elicit the onset of attack in an allergy-related asthma bronchial and conversely, the asthma-bronchial illness of a child can affect the rest of the family. A sibling may develop, for example, anorexia nervosa to claim his share of attention; the mother suffers a depressive crisis because the stress is too great.

Example 2: "Ulcus Duodeni" Ulcus duodeni was understood until 20 years ago as the consequence of stress and specific personality traits, such as passivity and dependence. With the discovery of the *Helicobacter pylori,* a somatic explanation was found for the occurrence and chronification of ulcus duodeni and its eradication by antibiotics. In fact, 60 % of people over 60 years of age are *H. pylori*-positive, of whom only 2 % develop an ulcus duodeni. That an ulcus duodeni may develop from the infection may also have a psychosocial cause.

K. Fritzsche (✉)
Department of Psychosomatic Medicine and Psychotherapy, University Medical Center, Hauptstr. 8, 79104 Freiburg, Germany
e-mail: kurt.fritzsche@uniklinik-freiburg.de

K. Fritzsche et al. (eds.), *Psychosomatic Medicine,* DOI 10.1007/978-1-4614-1022-5_1,

Example 3: "Coronary Heart Disease" Congenital and acquired dispositions and risk factors, elicitors ("Why now?"), and maintaining factors influence one another: coronary heart diseases in the family, cardiovascular risk factors like smoking, elevated blood lipids, hypertension, fear of losing one's job, partnership conflict with acute irritation, vital exhaustion, lack of social support, and depression.

The Biopsychosocial Model

Physical, emotional, and social factors in different proportions play a role in every illness. The doctor's task is to recognize not only the organic components, but also the psychosocial processes involved in the disease and to take these into account. Whether psychosocial stress is present can be clarified by the doctor only in the framework of a psychosocial anamnesis.

Case Study, continued While talking in the evening, the ward's doctor first sets the stage for the discussion: He had now about 15 min and would like to find out some information on the health and life history of the patient. The patient tells the following: Her father was killed in the war, she has no memories of him. The mother was overwhelmed with raising the patient and a younger and an older sister and had become an alcoholic. She moved to her grandmother whom she had experienced as very strict and emotionally cold. At the age of 23, she married and bore two daughters. Over the course of the marriage, the husband was increasingly becoming an alcoholic and died later of cirrhosis of the liver. The patient had separated in time, however. With a new partner, she opened a restaurant. This partnership also failed. The restaurant was carried on by her daughters and was closed down later. Last year, the older sister was diagnosed with cancer and died shortly thereafter. The patient has now taken over the care of her sister's son who is completely paraplegic.

(to be continued)

Bonding Experience

The life history of the patient is characterized by negative bonding experiences.

In healthy development, there is constant balancing between the attachment and the exploratory behavior (Fig. 1.1). Bonding behavior is activated in discomfort and stress, exploration behavior in well-being. *Bonding research* confirms the importance of early experiences for the physical and emotional health of a person. Uncertain, impaired early bonds decide whether a person can also withstand serious stress (*resilience*) or become ill (*vulnerability*). The first 3 years of life are decisive for bonding experiences.

If the infant or small child has a mother or another main reference person who responds *sensitively* with mimicry and gestures, that is quickly and appropriately to

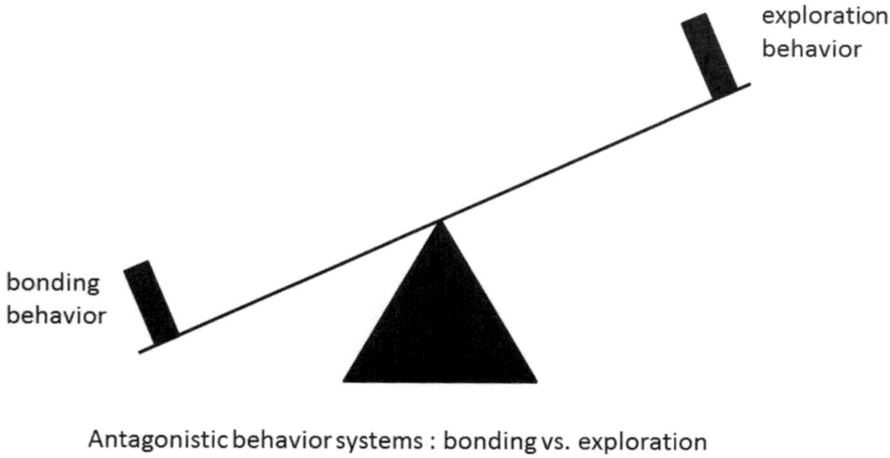

Fig. 1.1 Bonding versus exploration

the child's reactions, oxytocin is excreted, which enables the infant to experience social interactions and their attendant feelings as pleasant. A *secure bonding behavior* is promoted in this way. The brain, especially the amygdala, the hippocampus, and the prefrontal cortex are protected against damage in consequence of excessive glucocorticoid excretions in stress situations. Secure bonding contributes to an elevation of the stress threshold and dampening of the stress response. If, on the other hand, the mother reacts with rejection to the child's bonding needs, the result is a very *insecure-avoidant* bonding style in the child. If the maternal responses to the childish signals are contradictory and unpredictable, the child develops so-called *insecure-ambivalent* bonding.

Psychosocial Stress

A mother who suffers serious depression after the birth of her child cannot respond adequately to the child's bonding needs or empathize sufficiently with the child's needs. The lack of such *sensitivity* leads later to impairments in the development of the stress-coping system. Activation of the hypothalamus-pituitary-adrenal cortex (HPA) axis by increased corticotropin-releasing hormone (CRH) excretions or a lack of inhibition leads to increased cortisol and resultant damage to the hippocampus. Children who suffer great physical or emotional trauma develop hyperreactivity of the HPA and locus coeruleus-norepinephrine (LC-NE) axes. Psychosocial stress in childhood may thus lead to a dysfunction of the stress-coping system with elevated stress vulnerability in conflict situations.

Stress denotes the state of a threatened biological homeostasis or allostasis, which can be caused by both physical damage and by psychosocial burdens. Stress response or stress reaction is the body's attempt to reinstate biological homeostasis or allostasis

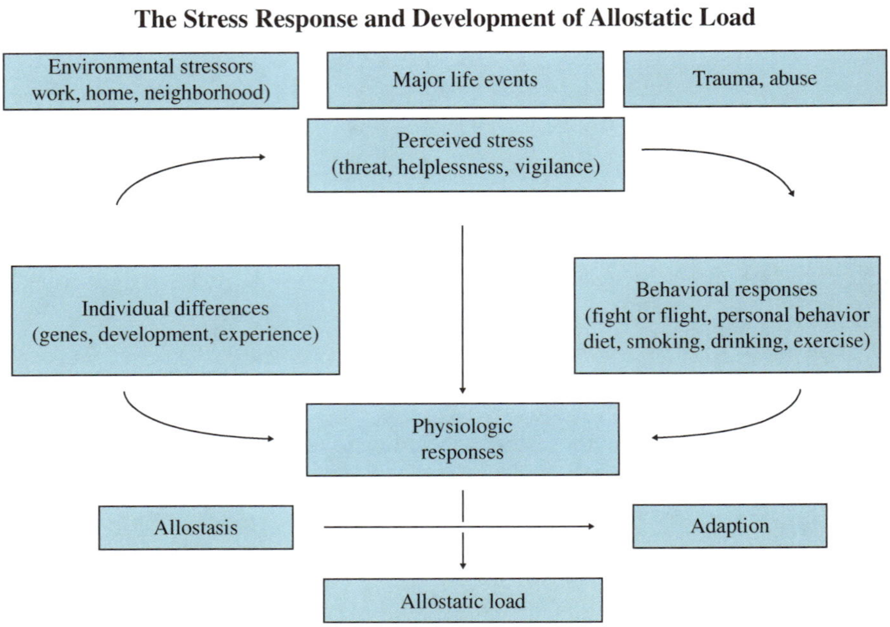

Fig. 1.2 The stress response and development of allostatic load (McEwen 1998)

by means of change and adaptation processes at the neuronal and endocrine levels and in behavior (Fig. 1.2). When the stress is over, the adaptation processes are inactivated again (McEwen 1998).

Case Study, continued The development of thrombosis with embolization in the right leg, developing gangrene at the right toe, poor wound healing, and recurrent infections may have been an expression of allostatic overload. In addition, there is increased stress vulnerability due to negative childhood experiences.

(to be continued)

Psyche and the Immune system

The death of a life partner, separation, or divorce leads to temporary loneliness, depression, and anxiety that, as stressors, affect the immune system. The immune system sends feedback to the nervous system in the form of cytokines. As part of an infection, they activate the HPA axis in order to curb the infection-induced immune activation. This produces the familiar feeling of illness in the form of fatigue, pain, loss of appetite, and body aches.

Overall, stress can promote, as well as suppress, the immune system. Short-term stress responses enhance the innate immune response. Satisfactory interpersonal relationships, physical well-being, and personal valuations strengthen the immune system. Permanent psychosocial stress such as job loss or loss of significant others, an accident with long-term consequences, chronic anger, or a chronic condition results in a reduction of T-lymphocytes, reducing the activity of natural killer cells, monocytes, and macrophages.

Example: "Autoimmune Diseases" The nervous system, endocrine system, and immune system form a unit. When one system does not respond adequately to a stressor, another system responds in the form of counter-regulation. If, for example, the cortisol excretion is no longer possible in response to a stressor, the inflammatory parameters like cytokine, which is normally inhibited by cortisone, increase in compensation. The negative consequence of a persistent excessive inflammatory response is a greater susceptibility to autoimmune diseases. Examples of reactions to underregulation on the HPA axis are patients with fibromyalgia, chronic fatigue syndrome or patients with atopic dermatitis.

Learning Experience and Cognitions

In *cognitions,* fundamental convictions and assumptions about one's self and the world are especially important. Every person has certain basic convictions, so-called patterns. These patterns have their origin in early childhood relationship experiences and are further formed later by cultural and family influences as well as personal experiences. The focus of the cognitive theory is the assumption that the patient's convictions are important to his behavior, his emotions, and also his physical reactions.

Example: Learning Experiences "Suppression of Emotions" Many patients have learned from a family climate in which feelings and conflicts are not expressed, and irritation, rage, disappointment, and sadness are not even perceived. The affects go "inward," they activate the attendant psychophysiological processes, whereby the patient appears passive and withdrawn on the surface. The psychophysiological reactions lead, however, to an activation of the HPA axis with increased cortisone excretion, inhibition of the immune system, and activation of its back-coupling processes to the central nervous system. Suppression of emotional experience and the related initial avoidance of conflicts has a transient relief function, but in the long term, it promotes the occurrence of anxiety and depression, physical complaints without organ findings up to and including chronic pain states.

Case Study, continued For her, the hospital situation means a reactivation of early childhood loneliness and abandonment. She is admitted because of a harmless lesion and then experiences one unsuccessful intervention after another, until finally an amputation of the right lower leg becomes necessary. She was accustomed to fighting and getting back on her feet. This path seems now cut off. The ward doctor understands that the patient had always lived caring for others, and now suddenly feels left alone with no prospects. He summarizes the conversation in his own words, showing his emotional understanding and assures that he will be there for her. The patient feels relieved after the conversation, and can again smile a bit, and with adequate pain medication spends a quiet night.

(to be continued)

Salutogenesis and Resilience

Case Study, continued The further course is uneventful. The medical history interview revealed that the patient, despite the current hopelessness, has good resources of her own in terms of fighting spirit and social skills. After a period of mourning over the loss of the leg, she is very actively involved in the mobilization. The adaptation of a prosthesis is achieved without difficulty. The patient wants to go for the rehabilitation in a hospital that has been offered. Three weeks later at discharge, the patient is again cautiously optimistic regarding her future and is very grateful for the professional and emotional support by the ward doctor. The ward doctor also feels appreciated for his effort and relieved.

Whether a person becomes ill depends on the interactions between stress factors and protective factors. Protective factors can offset the negative experiences in the child's development and lead to strengthening of the emotional *resilience*. Since the neuronal linking in the brain is immediately related to the rearing and socialization which the child experiences in the first 3 years of life, deficits in brain development can also be offset in this way.

In researching the *development of health* (salutogenesis), Antonovsky (1987) sought conditions which enable a person to remain physically and emotionally healthy in difficult life situations, such as death of a close person, an accident or an emotional crisis, or to regain health. By examining holocaust survivors, Antonovsky reached the conviction that salutogenesis depends on a *sense of coherence*, that is, stressful life events can be comprehended, managed, and are meaningful. Antonovsky considers the *sense of coherence* a basic, life-preserving resource, which the person develops during his life by coping with and overcoming problems. *Resource activation* connects to the patient's positive characteristics, capabilities, and motivations in organizing his life and his interpersonal relationships.

Sense of coherence includes the capability of:

- Experiencing stressful events as comprehensible (*Comprehensibility*)
- Managing these events (*Manageability*)
- Attributing to such stress meaning and sense (*Meaningfulness*)

Epigenetics

Psychosomatic connections are also found in the regulation of gene activity. Psychological and psychosomatic disorders and problems are often based on the empirically proven fact that interpersonal relationship experiences affect the activity of specific neurobiologically relevant genes and may alter epigenetic patterns, i.e., the long-term readability of genes. This also applies to long-term negative relationship experiences and traumas. The DNA sequence remains the same, the activity of genes, however, is changed significantly. As a consequence, functionality of the brain and other organs may be affected and psychosomatic disorders are triggered.

Studies show that addictions, depression, and certain types of behavior are associated with epigenetic modifications of neurobiologically relevant genes. There is preliminary evidence that these epigenetic changes can also be hereditary. Specifically, it was shown in animal experiments that in pups of mothers caring little for them, the regulatory sequences of the gene for the glucocorticoid receptor were increasingly methylated in the offspring. Methylation means that the activity of a DNA section is inhibited. This increased methylation was detected in the hippocampus, among other things, a brain region that is important for learning and memory. The affected nerve cells produced less receptor molecules and this increased, in particular, the stress response of the animals. Even as adults, the affected pups were more anxious and could be upset more easily. This effect lasted for life. It is clear that, particularly early environmental influences and interpersonal relationship experiences, especially traumatic experiences, can alter the regulation of epigenetic gene structures.

Cultural Aspects

See Chap. 4 "Traditional Medicine and Psychosomatic Medicine"

References

Antonovsky A. The salutogenetic perspective: Toward a new view of health and illness. Advances. 1987; 4:47–55.

McEwen BS. Protective and demaging effects of stress mediators. New Engl. J Med. 1998; 338:171–179.

Chapter 2
Psychosomatic Medicine in Primary Care

Kurt Fritzsche

The theoretical basis of Psychosomatic Medicine is the biopsychosocial model system (Engel 1977). This system describes the interactions among the biological, psychological, and social processes that are involved, to different extents, in each disease. In many Western countries, basic knowledge about recognizing psychological and psychosomatic disorders and problems, counseling and providing emotional support, and providing referrals to health specialists are included in the training of medical students and postgraduate doctors. The objectives of the psychosomatic approach are to build bridges between the various clinical disciplines to overcome the mind–body dichotomy and to stress the importance of understanding the interactions among biology, psychology, and social factors in every patient, independent of the primary pathology that is being treated. These objectives imply both a system-based perspective and knowledge of the biological, psychological, and social subsystems and their interactions. The psychosomatic approach focuses on the doctor–patient relationship and on an integrative strategy for diagnosing and treating patients. Educating and training the somatic clinician to integrate psychosomatic aspects of medical care into his/her daily work has become a well-accepted priority for training and research.

Psychosomatic Medicine in primary care has primarily been influenced by psychoanalysts and internists who emulated Balint's (1964) approach, which stressed the integration of psychosomatic and holistic perspectives in the medical practice model.

This integrated biopsychosocial treatment includes the following advantages:

1. The physical examination is integrated into the consulting hour. Beginning with the patient's presentation of complaints, the doctor assesses both somatic and emotional concerns. As a result, both physical and psychosocial problems are addressed in diagnosis and treatment.

K. Fritzsche (✉)
Department of Psychosomatic Medicine and Psychotherapy, University Medical Center, Hauptstr. 8, Freiburg 79104, Germany
e-mail: kurt.fritzsche@uniklinik-freiburg.de

K. Fritzsche et al. (eds.), *Psychosomatic Medicine,* DOI 10.1007/978-1-4614-1022-5_2,

2. Many patients do not feel as embarrassed about conversations regarding mental or interpersonal conflicts in the primary care setting as they might if referred to a mental health professional.
3. Conversations in the primary care setting usually occur in the context of long-standing, trusting doctor–patient relationships. Such relationships have been shown to be important factors in the healing process. Family conflicts and past crises are usually familiar to the doctor who treats the entire family. When a new conflict or symptom arises, it can be placed in a personalized context.

References

Balint M. The doctor, his patient and the illness. 2nd ed. London: Pitman; 1964. (3rd Millennium edition: Edinburgh: Churchill Livingstone; 2000).

Engel GL. The need for a new medical model: a challenge for biomedicine. Science. 1977;196: 129–136.

Chapter 3
Objectives of Training in Psychosomatic Medicine in Primary Care

Kurt Fritzsche

The four targeted skills of Psychosomatic Medicine in primary care include the following:

1. Identifying stressful emotional and mental disorders and conflicts using a psychosocial anamnesis
2. Promoting a helping alliance among the doctor, patient, and family members; this skill also includes identifying possible barriers on the part of the doctor, patient, or family and stressing the core skills of empathy and sensitivity
3. Improving the patient's problem-solving skills, including providing information about self-help groups, supporting the management of adverse life events (e.g., severe illness, loss, separation, or divorce) and avoiding unnecessary medication, diagnostic procedures, and surgery
4. Motivating/referring patients for psychotherapy. Additional skills in this area include collaborations around consultations and case management with psychotherapists and other psychosocial service providers.

Targeted Skill 1: Disease Patterns

The selection of mental disease to be taught depends on the frequencies of the diseases' occurrences in different countries. The following diseases have been deemed important: (1) the various forms of depression; (2) anxiety disorders (3) somatoform disorders; (4) adjustment disorders to severe life-threatening diseases, such as cancer and coronary heart disease; (5) posttraumatic stress disorder (PTSD); (6) alcohol, drug, and internet addiction. Psychopharmacological treatment approaches have been integrated into the education about each disease pattern.

K. Fritzsche (✉)
Department of Psychosomatic Medicine and Psychotherapy, University Medical Center, Hauptstr. 8, 79104 Freiburg, Germany
e-mail: kurt.fritzsche@uniklinik-freiburg.de

K. Fritzsche et al. (eds.), *Psychosomatic Medicine*, DOI 10.1007/978-1-4614-1022-5_3,

Targeted Skills 2 and 3: Interventions

The basic therapeutic approaches integrate psychodynamic approaches, cognitive-behavioral models, systemic family therapy, and communication skills, such as empathy, unconditional positive regard, and congruence, to develop good doctor–patient relationships (Rogers 1997). Examples of the use of cognitive-behavioral models include the vicious circle model in the area of anxiety disorders and the influence of negative thinking and avoidant behaviors in depression. In the treatment of patients with somatoform disorders, the disease model of the patient, which has traditionally focused on physical causes, is gradually expanded to include alternative concepts of illness, and the attention is refocused on potential psychosocial stressors. In systemic thinking, interactions replace reductionist notions of cause and effect.

The teaching of doctor–patient communication skills includes learning interview techniques that are both doctor centered and patient centered, allowing time for the patient to talk at the beginning of the interview, not interrupting, asking open questions, offering verbal and nonverbal encouragement to keep talking, summarizing in your own words, and reflecting emotions.

An ideal method for understanding doctor–patient interactions is the Balint group, in which the focus is placed on difficult interactions between doctor and patient.

Targeted Skill 4: Collaboration with Mental Health Specialists

The fourth learning objective involves referrals to mental health specialists and cooperation with mental health services. Even in Western countries with well-developed support systems, these processes are not optimal. Primary care physicians have an important pilot function in the mental health-care system. They must decide whether basic psychosomatic care is sufficient or expert assistance should be requested, as well as which expert is best suited to address the problem. The primary care physician should inform the patient of the need for more intensive psychotherapeutic and/or psychopharmacological treatment, should motivate him/her to accept such an offer and should refer him/her to the appropriate physician or facilities.

References

Rogers CR. Empathic: an unappreciated way of being. Couns Psychol. 1997;5:2–10.

Chapter 4
Traditional Medicine and Psychosomatic Medicine

Kurt Fritzsche, Catherine Abbo, Hamid Afshar Zanjani and Farzad Goli

Traditional Chinese Medicine

Traditional Chinese medicine (TCM) is one of the oldest healing systems. Most of the principles of TCM derived from the philosophical basis that contributed to the development of Taoism and Confucianism. The goal is that natural phenomena could be categorized into yin and yang. Everything in the universe consisted of five basic elements (wood, fire, earth, metal, and water) and the universe was constantly changing toward dynamic balance or harmony. Such knowledge was applied to understand, prevent, and cure disease.

TCM includes herbal medicine, acupuncture, moxibustion, massage, food therapy, and physical exercise such as shadow boxing). It is estimated that 40 % of health care in China is based on TCM, with a higher proportion in rural areas. Every city has a hospital practicing TCM, and there is a plan for every county to have one.

K. Fritzsche (✉)
Department of Psychosomatic Medicine and Psychotherapy,
University Medical Center, Hauptstr. 8, 79104 Freiburg, Germany
e-mail: kurt.fritzsche@uniklinik-freiburg.de

C. Abbo
Department of Psychiatry, Makerere University College
of Health Sciences and Mulago National Referral and Teaching Hospital,
Mulago Hill Road, Kampala 7072, Uganda
e-mail: cathyabbo@chs.mak.ac.ug, cathya180@gmail.com

H. Afshar Zanjani
Department of Psychiatry, Medical Faculty, Psychosomatic Research Center,
Isfahan University of Medical Sciences, Noor Hospital, 5th Fl, Baghbeh Bld.,
36th Alley, Tohid St., Shariati St, 48763-81739, Isfahan, 81736-44165 Isfahan, Iran
e-mail: afshar@med.mui.ac.ir, shafsharz@gmail.com

F. Goli
Department of bioenergy economy,
Energy Medicine University, California, USA
e-mail: Dr.fgoli@yahoo.com

Danesh-e Tandorosti Institute, Isfahan, Iran
e-mail: info@iranianhealth.com

K. Fritzsche et al. (eds.), *Psychosomatic Medicine,* DOI 10.1007/978-1-4614-1022-5_4,

In 95 % of hospitals practicing Western medicine, there are departments of TCM, most with patient beds. When patients arrive at the outpatient department they can opt for Chinese or Western treatment. In Western medicine hospitals, around 40 % of medicines prescribed are traditional. Herbs are used much more commonly then acupuncture (Tang et al. 2008).

Disease occurs after a disturbance in yin-yang, or flow of qi, or blood, or disharmony in the organs caused by personage (e.g., sadness, joy, and lifestyle) and climatic factors (dampness, heat, cold). Treatment aims to expel or suppress the cause and restore balance.

The integration of TCM in Western medicine has been widely promoted and studied in China and in Western countries. Integration aims eventually to combine these two systems. Currently, integration is mainly at the level of physicians who have received training and can treat patients in both. For example, over a third of the training in TCM schools is in Western medicine, and Western-medicine schools also offer some training in TCM.

Research is needed to determine which illnesses are best treated by one approach rather than the other. In China, Western medicine is often regarded as more effective in an acute situation or where the etiology is known, while TCM is more effective for immune conditions, chronic illness, or where the etiology is unknown.

Psychosomatic Aspects in TCM

TCM has a holistic view of body and mind and the acceptance of somatic presentation of emotion is common. This is parallel to modern psychosomatic approaches (Tseng 2001). The heart was thought to house the superior mind, the liver to control spiritual soul, the lungs, the animal soul, the spleen ideas and intelligence, and the kidney vitality and will.

When vital air was concentrated on the heart, joy was created; on the lungs, sorrow; on the liver, anger; on the spleen, worry; on the kidney, fear. Thus, it was considered that various emotions were stirred through the visceral organs. In accordance with this medical knowledge in daily life, many organ-related sayings were used by the common people such as "elevated liver fire," "loosing spleen spirit," "hasty heart," "angry liver," or "exhausted kidney," to denote emotional state.

TCM has some advantages in the treatment of psychological and psychosomatic symptoms:

1. Patients prefer a more holistic view of their illness and do not encourage separation in physical and psychological causes.
2. Even if patients are aware of the psychosocial stress being an underlying cause of their condition, they rather opt for a more somatically oriented way to describe and treat their symptoms.
3. Patients expect from doctors that they will ask them about their physical symptoms, perform a physical exam, and take their pulse. They feel uncomfortable when doctors ask them about psychosocial aspects of their illness.

Ayurvedic Medicine

The term "Ayurveda" comes from the Indian Sanskrit and is composed of the words *Ayus* (life) and *Veda* (knowledge). Ayurveda claims a holistic approach in that human health and disease are seen as the interplay of physical, mental, emotional, and spiritual aspects (Kutumbiah 1962).

Different temperaments or vital energies called *Doshas* are distinguished:

- *Vata* (wind, air, and aether), the concept of movement
- *Pitta* (fire and water), the concept of fire and metabolism
- *Kapha* (earth and water), the concept of structure

In a healthy organism, the *Doshas* should exist in a harmonious equilibrium. The doctor determines the current relationship between the *Doshas* by means of pulse diagnosis and from the patient's astrological horoscope. To balance the *Doshas* and to drain accumulated waste, certain cleaning procedures (*Panchakarma*) are employed. These *Panchakarma* include fasting, baths, enemas, vomiting, and bloodletting, and also massages, yoga, and breathing exercises, color and music therapy, and the use of Ayurvedic medicines.

The goal of Ayurvedic medicine is to prevent serious diseases by trying to understand the cause of the disease and to eliminate unhealthy habits. The diagnosis is made by a whole-body examination including pulse and urine tests, and an examination of tongue and eyes.

Ayurvedic medicine includes a special dietetics. Food is considered to be information for the *Doshas*. Ideally, this information is converted into *Ojas*, an intangible superfine substance that is also produced when making positive experiences. *Ojas* strengthens the body's natural defenses and connects body and mind.

Diseases are divided into three groups: physical, accidental, and mental. *Physical disease* arises from abnormal conditions of the body. *Accidental diseases* are caused by the action of spirits, poisons, wind, fire, and violence the body experiences. *Mental diseases* are caused by unsatisfied basic emotional needs. Pronounced anger, sadness, fear, and anxiety are an expression of a mental imbalance. It is clearly apparent that emotional distress is recognized as a cause of disease. In addition to treatment with herbs and drugs, Ayurvedic medicine includes a detailed description of psychotherapeutic techniques for the treatment of mental disorders.

Mental health is seen as an integral part of life. Firmly rooted is also the notion that emotional ties, love, and affection of closely related persons are just as or even more effective in the treatment of mental disorders as doctors and their treatment methods.

Possibly, parts of the Ayurvedic theory and some drug preparations have been adopted from the Greek medicine. In Plato's system, health is based on a harmonic balance between the three elements *Pneuma* (air or *Vata*), *Chole* (bile or *Pitta*), and *Phlegm* (mucus, fire, or *Kapha*). The Greek medicine on the other hand has influenced the Galenic-Islamic medicine.

Ayurveda got lost almost completely with the fall of the Vedic culture. Only in Sri Lanka, it is applied consistently even to date. Sri Lanka is the only country that offers state-funded Ayurveda as a complete health-care system. In India, too, Ayurveda still plays a role in health care, although to a lesser extent. In many Western countries, Ayurveda is used as an alternative and complementary medicine.

Islamic Medicine in Iran

In Iranian traditional medicine there were three schools of medicine: methodism, empiricism, and dogmatism. The *methodists* focused on symptomatic treatment and they did not care about etiology and pathology. The *empiricists* claimed that management plans should be obtained through experience and concrete observation. They emphasized a disease-oriented approach and believed that each therapy which had-been effective in a patient evidently would be effective for other patients with the same disease. This school of medicine is the grandfather of modern biomedicine. The *dogmatists* held that there was no doubt that sense and experience were the facts, but they had to be derived through thought and analogy. In spite of the empiricists, the dogmatists did not believe in generalization of management plans to all cases of a disease. In addition to signs and symptoms, and nosological classifications, dogmatists carefully mentioned illness experiences, individual differences, humoral and psychological states, family support, and occupational and environmental parameters in their management (Ibne-I Hindu 1989). Evidently, this approach is a precursor of Psychosomatic Medicine.

The traditional medicine of Iran is based on Unani medicine, and was developed by the great physicians of the Middle Ages such as Razi (865–925), Ibn-e Sina (Avicenna) (980–1037), and Jorjani (1042–1137). Like most of the comprehensive traditional medicine systems, it relied on the concept of “equilibrium” of nonlocal natural forces and qualities (humors; Bannerman and Bannerman 1983). Disease is defined as an imbalanced outcome of internal/external forces. Treatment in this approach is not focused on the removal or alternating of the local pathogenesis but is organized around managing the natural forces of the body and environment.

There is no dualistic border between mental and physical illness in this healing system, and both of them are analyzed as systemic imbalance of the natural forces, and *Psyche* is nothing but the function of the *Soma* which can act independently and is autogenous in some way.

The “Health Calendar” of Ibn-e Botlan (2003) is a typical sample of this world-view. Each person, illness, part of the body, food, remedy, mental or physical activity, time, place, color, and order has its special temperament and we should conduct these natural forces prudently into our life to maintain and promote our dynamic equilibrium of the forces.

For maintaining and promoting of mental health in Iranian traditional medicine, you should recognize first the temper of the brain and then the temper of the disorder, then you can manage the health condition. For example, a person with warm and wet brain is supposed to be prone to headache and nightmare. Their wits are not so blunt, they sleep deep and long, and they have difficulties in obtaining and retaining information. So, wet and warm foods, remedies, and weather resonates this trend. Furthermore, in this system each disorder has its own specific nature (Ibn-e Botlan 2003). For example, it is believed that two main deviations from a normal and balanced brain are: anxiety-restlessness and depression-weakness; the first one arouses from excessive warmness and/or dryness and the second one is because of coldness and/or wetness of the brain (Jorjani 1966).

Phobia, worry, impulsivity, and paranoia signify warmness of brain and it is supposed that we should manage these conditions by cold-tempered foods, drinks, remedies, mental and physical activities. One of the ways in which we can diagnose the brain temperament is by dream analysis. For instance the dominant color of dream signifies dominant humor; red spectrum is induced by blood, yellow by bile, and white by phlegm.

Religious and Spiritual Healing in Africa

In most African societies, healing goes beyond the alleviation of individual history and includes mending of social divisions which exist both within and between communities. Health is traditionally defined as harmonious relationships between human beings and their natural surroundings, and between them and their ancestors, and among themselves.

The social world (comprising the spirits and the living) and the physical world are united within a larger cosmology. If this harmonious state breaks down, it is seen as a result of malevolent intervention or a sanction by the ancestors for incorrect or inappropriate social behavior. Although a large proportion of Africans have converted to Islam and Christianity, these two world religions have been assimilated into African culture, and many African Christians and Muslims maintain traditional spiritual beliefs. Furthermore, African cultural practices contain elements of indigenous religion. Thus, traditional African cosmologies and beliefs continue to exert significant influence on Africans today. The power of spiritual entities remains paramount in the causation and treatment of mental disorders. It is by means of spiritual understanding that people can restore meaning and sense of balance to their lives following traumatic experiences (see chapter about PTSD). Appeasing the spirits for example, is thus a mechanism for redressing the wrongs of the past and restoring well-being.

Religious/spiritual practices that can be of benefit to the health worker's medical practice and well-being:

- Open prayer (ecumenical prayer): This can be held with clients in the patients' waiting room each morning before formal treatment begins
- Personal reflection (on personal life, life of others, nature)
- Promotion of humanitarian service (give back to humanity)
- Forgiveness of Self-Forgiveness
- Acceptance that some of the problems are beyond you and that you need to surrender them to a "higher being"

- Adaption of some of the spiritual rituals/practices such as singing and dancing
- Undertaking physical exercise and self-care
- Promotion of positivism, self-efficacy, and self-actualization

Attitudes Toward Indigenous Healing Practices

Some medical doctors see folk healing as merely "superstitious" and "primitive," insisting that such out-of-date practices should be discouraged or prohibited. Other doctors consider these folk practices to be interesting subjects for academic study. They want to examine the therapeutic elements that they utilize and why such supernaturally orientated therapeutic exercises are still popular among some groups. Other doctors or community health workers believe that due to shortage of professional personnel available in the community, the existence of "Folk" therapies should be supported (Tseng 2001). The joint declaration on primary health care made in 1978 by the World Health Organization and the UNICEF at Alma Ata, Kazakhstan gave international recognition to the positive role of indigenous practitioners. Any folk healing practice that is proven to be helpful to the client and useful to the community deserves the support and encouragement of clinicians as well as administrators. The collaboration of indigenous healers and modern clinicians should be encouraged to provide maximal mental health services for the community.

Cultural Responsibility

Every physician should be "culturally responsible" when dealing with a patient with emotional problems from a different cultural background. Cultural responsibility starts with cultural competence—that is, one's ability to work with people of different cultural backgrounds. Cultural responsibility means going beyond cultural competence and taking responsibility for the way we view culture. It means that people of all cultural backgrounds work together respectfully and effectively with knowledge and awareness. It includes attitudes, behaviors, skills, policies, and procedures.

Cultural responsibility might include:

- Understanding and/or learning from the cultural group you are dealing with
- Building links between health services and culture-based community organizations or other organizations that serve a specific community, and recognizing the experiences and expertise of cultural organizations and leaders in our communities
- Providing helpful, tailored information in a language that is understood by the patient
- Recognizing the role of cultural, medical, or health practices
- Considering importance of religion and spirituality in the management and treatment of mental disorders

- Considering extended family network in the management and treatment of mental disorders
- Looking at the whole person beyond cultural or any other borders
- Looking at the bigger picture and recognizing that it is difficult to separate mental problems from larger concerns, like poverty or lack of housing

Summary

All medical tradition had its origin in a religious world view, which assigned Gods the power to afflict illness on people. During the fifth century before Christ, Greek medicine tried to understand illnesses based on the laws of nature. The teachings of the four elements and the four humors were created and an independent medical science developed therefrom. The basis of all life is an equal interconnectedness of four elements or basic substances: fire, water, air, and earth. Any living being and the entire universe are made of them. This holistic perspective shows parallels to Chinese medicine, to Ayurveda, and the Persian Islamic medicine. It is obvious that there has been a far-reaching cross-cultural parallelism of traditions for more than two millennia. In addition, medical science is closely tied to the societal and economic conditions of life and how people view life. Just like Paul Unschuld interpreted it in his book *What is Medicine? Western and Eastern Approaches to Healing* (Unschuld 2009).

Over millennia, the knowledge of the power of the Gods, our ancestors and demons have largely determined human actions in all cultures. This type of thought was alive and is alive parallel to the development of modern life sciences.

Many ideas of holistic medicine are found until this day in the home remedies and folk medicine of Western countries. There are departments for natural healing at universities. Additional study programs are offered in homeopathy and an independent approach to healing that is based on a religious world view such as the medical anthroposophic medicine.

References

Bannerman IARC, Bannerman RH. Traditional medicine and health care coverage: a reader for health administrators and practitioners. Geneva: World Health Organization; 1983.

Ibn-e Botlan B. In: Yosefi GH, Editor. Taghvim al Sehat. Tehran; 2003. [farsi].

Ibne-I Hindu AF. In: Mohaghegh M, Daneshpajuh MT, editors. Miftah al-Tibb wa-Minhaj al-Tullab. Tehran: Mc Gill University in collaboration with Tehran University; 1989. pp. 33–48.

Jorjani SE. Al-Aghraz al Tibbia val Mabahess al-Alaiia. Bonyad-e Farhang-e Iran, Tehran, 1966. [farsi].

Kutumbiah P. Ancient Indian medicine. Calcutta: Orient Longmans; 1962.

Tang JL, Liu BY, Ma KW. Traditional Chinese medicine. Lancet. 2008;372:1938–40.

Tseng WS. Handbook of cultural psychiatry. San Diego: Academic press; 2001.

Unschuld PU. What is medicine? Western and eastern approaches to healing. Berkeley: University of California Press; 2009.

Part II
The First Contact—Basic Interventions

Chapter 5
The Doctor–Patient Relationship

Kurt Fritzsche, Catherine Abbo, Gertrud Frahm and Sonia Diaz Monsalve

A trustworthy relationship between doctor and patient that is experienced as helpful forms the foundation of any medical treatment. The doctor is the only one with regular and frequent encounters of conflicts, fears and needs, which burden people of all age groups, social classes and nationalities as a result or cause of physical or mental suffering. The quality of the doctor–patient relationship is the decisive factor for the success of treatment. Doctors combining empathy with assured demeanor and understandable information have better treatment outcomes compared to doctors with a more impersonal, formal, or unclear appearance.

Every doctor has had the experience that he himself or she herself does more good for the sick than a medicine. The perception and handling of the doctor himself/herself as a drug is a key task in dealing with patients. The doctor tries to understand how the patient's behavior affects his/her reactions and vice versa. This division of attention between dealing with the patient and his/her own emotional reactions and their impact on the physician's own behavior is something very unusual, which requires patience, concentration, and constant training. The doctor himself/herself facilitates to a great extent, or not, whether the patient will be able to open up, talk about himself/herself or whether he/she is withdrawing and provides only monosyllabic answers to questions (Balint 2000).

K. Fritzsche (✉) · S. D. Monsalve
Department of Psychosomatic Medicine and Psychotherapy,
University Medical Center, Hauptstr. 8, 79104 Freiburg, Germany
e-mail: kurt.fritzsche@uniklinik-freiburg.de

S. D. Monsalve
e-mail: sonia.diaz-monsalve@uniklinik-freiburg.de

C. Abbo
Department of Psychiatry, Makerere University College
of Health Sciences and Mulago National Referral and Teaching Hospital,
Mulago Hill Road, 7072 Kampala, Uganda
e-mail: cathyabbo@chs.mak.ac.ug, cathya180@gmail.com

G. Frahm
Department of Human Sciences, Federal University of Paraná,
R. Gal. Carneiro, 460, Curitiba, PR 80060-150, Brazil
e-mail: gfrahm@uol.com.br

K. Fritzsche et al. (eds.), *Psychosomatic Medicine*, DOI 10.1007/978-1-4614-1022-5_5,

Forms of the Doctor–Patient Relationship

Because of their roles, and the physician's fund of knowledge and training, the relationship between doctor and patient is and will remain asymmetric at the core. The asymmetry intensifies because of rapid advances in medicine, but it reduces by new information sources (Internet) and in patients with high level of education. Therefore, the doctor needs to be highly flexible and must have a very good feel for the individual patient.

The Paternalistic Model

The paternalistic model arises from Hippocratic thinking. Accordingly, the doctor, by virtue of his (paternal) authority, is in a position to make decisions for the patient (who is deemed incompetent), for the benefit of the patient, and to act on them. Here the doctor knows as a medical expert, what is best for the patient. He/she violates the autonomy of the patient, based on the conviction that this is happening to the patient's benefit.

In the conversation between doctor and patient, the doctor determines the topics that are being talked about. The interview is used to query diagnostic criteria that cannot be directly observed by examination. It focuses on somatic findings. Often, the complaints are registered through closed or standardized questions. In this model, the doctor may be guided optimally by the best scientific standards when treating a patient. He/she contributes and his/her expertise and suggestions for treatment are based on medical expertise. The patient is merely told about the treatment that is derived from the findings. The compliance of the patient with medical instructions is assumed.

Case study "36-year-old patient in cardiac ambulance to discuss findings"
A: According to the findings, it is a high degree aortic stenosis which absolutely requires surgery within the next few weeks. I already scheduled an admission date at the surgical clinic for 02/13. In the meantime, please refrain from any physical activity. Continue to take your medication. After surgery, you will be staying in the intensive care unit. When in stable condition, you will move to the floor. Subsequently, we will request a rehabilitation therapy.

This approach has advantages, but it also disadvantages which are listed in Table 5.1.

The Service or Consumer Model

The medical care becomes a service, from which the claim is derived, to see the doctor as the service provider and the patient as the consumer. In this model, the doctor is an expert, the decision-making authority remains with the patient. The

Table 5.1 Advantages and disadvantages of the paternalistic model

Advantages	Disadvantages
Diagnosis is brief and calculable by closed questions	By focusing on somatic relationships additional diagnoses or other important information are overlooked
Irritations are avoided with additional information	Lack of compliance of patients. Some patients build confidence only then when they feel perceived and observed as a person and not just as a sick body
With definite diagnosis the patients get the best treatment in a short time	
Suitable for patients who expect a paternalistic doctor and come with great confidence in him	

physician's role is limited to providing the patient with the necessary information and to carry out the decisions taken by the patient. Since the doctor is liable for the treatment, the rules of medical science must be observed. Not everything that the "patient as the customer" may desire may be or has to be carried out by the doctor.

In the doctor–patient consultation patient satisfaction is paramount. The attitude of the patient is characterized by mistrust that the doctor is looking to overcome by friendly and expert advice. The doctor thus satisfies the needs of the patient for freedom, independence, being informed, and respectful attention. The patient has the right to make demands, the physician, however, should remain friendly even if the patient exaggerates.

Case study "61-year-old patient with severe aortic stenosis and aortic aneurysm"

A: I can tell that you are not thrilled about the news about a necessary surgery. I can assure you that we will operate carefully and with the utmost professionalism. Foregoing surgery, however, will involve a high risk that you would have to bear.

P: The scheduled date 3 weeks from now is too early. I'm traveling on business and would like to go on vacation afterwards. Can we reschedule the surgery for a later date?

A: This is difficult, according to the findings the surgery should be carried out soon. Of course, you can wait, in the meantime we reduce the risk with drugs, however, a significant risk remains that you would have to bear.

Advantages and disadvantages of this model are listed in Table 5.2.

The Partnership Model

The partnership model is based on the cooperative effort between two equal partners. Only if both work together and complement each other, the treatment can lead to a

Table 5.2 Advantages and disadvantages of the service model

Advantages	Disadvantages
Patient satisfaction; patient can talk about things that are not disease related	Risk of carrying out treatments which are not indicated
Doctor satisfies social needs to a greater extent	Often, the doctor must confront patients against their will with unpleasant but necessary decisions. The patient possibly turns to another doctor, who fulfills his/her wishes. Many patients expect emotional involvement
Compliance problems are rare	
People with severe need for autonomy are satisfied with this type of relationship	

Table 5.3 Advantages and disadvantages of the partnership model

Advantages	Disadvantages
Patient takes responsibility; compliance problems are avoided	Difficult task to inform the patient in a manner so that he/she will be able to take the responsibility
Doctor is relieved because he/she does not have to decide on difficult ethical questions	Takes a long time for medical history; unpaid additional effort requires idealism on the part of the doctor
Subsequent treatment shortened by building confidence	
Especially useful during prolonged monitoring of patients	

successful outcome. The patient is respected as a mature person who makes his life decisions autonomously (principle of autonomy). The doctor is the expert. His/her mission is to inform the patient so that he/she is capable of reasoned decision. In this model, the patient can, may, and should contribute his/her own questions and positions to the conversation with his doctor. They work together to find the best possible solution (shared decision making, see note). The patient has the right to refuse any treatment, if done in full awareness of the consequences of doing so. The doctor has to accept it. In this negotiation process, doctors and patients are collectively responsible for all decisions. This is true even if one or both had envisioned something different or considered something more desirable.

Case study "Coronary artery bypass grafting surgery"
A: I have shared with you the results and would now like to hear what your thoughts are and whether you agree with the decision of my colleagues.
P: For once I am shocked that I have to undergo surgery immediately; I would have preferred having a bit more time.
A: Yes, I see that the finding is very surprising to you and you must get used to the situation. I would be happy to explain once again the advantages of an early surgery.
P: Please go ahead.

Advantages and disadvantages of the partnership model are listed in Table 5.3.

The goal of shared decision making is a jointly supported decision of two, in principle, equal partners. To achieve this, both sides must be willing to come to a joint decision, to share relevant information and be willing to make a decision and accept it.

For the patient is important to obtain the following information:

- Basic information about the disease
- Information to get an idea about the prognosis
- Information to understand the course of examinations and treatments
- Information in order to be able to assess the consequences of examinations and treatments
- Ways of supporting
- Ways to avoid complications

The doctor may ask the patient to explain his/her decision in his/her own words. Supporting graphics can be used, which serve both the perceptual information and the clarification of risks.

It is the decision of each doctor to what extent he/she includes the models described in his/her professional identity. The partnership model requires the doctor to be highly flexible and to be able to listen. Psychological or social problems are often addressed only reluctantly and in disguised form. If the doctor does not notice the hints of patients, psychosocial issues are increasingly being excluded from the patient. The decision to walk the more difficult path of being more flexible toward the patient, will be rewarded long term with more grateful patients and increased job satisfaction.

Pitfalls

- In the implementation of the models one's own expectations about oneself can be too high. The attitudes described are ideals that can rarely be matched one-to-one. Therefore, go ahead and experiment with these models.
- The expectations of patients both for autonomy and trust and security are being considered too one-sided.

Cultural Aspects

General

While in much of the Western world, a family doctor is the first contact who, if necessary, will refer the patient to a specialist, "doctor shopping" takes place in many parts of the world. In case of dissatisfaction doctors will be switched or various practitioners will be consulted in parallel. This does not further sustainable care and may result in misdiagnosis. Depending on the cultural background, patients show different attitudes toward proposed treatments. Doctors should reflect on their own value system as well as that of their patients in order to be able to deal with possible deviations.

Asia

In the USA, a cooperative doctor–patient relationship, based predominantly on the values of individualism, autonomy, and service, is predominant. In contrast, in many Asian societies, the doctor–patient relationship is structured according to the model of a hierarchical relationship (Nilchaikovit et al. 1993). Here, the doctor is the virtuous authority figure, caring and responsible for the welfare of the patient. In return, he/she receives respect and deference. If an Asian patient is treated by an American doctor, it may result in cultural misunderstandings due to these different models, on which this encounter is based on. If, from the perspective of the patient, for example, certain expectations are not met, the patient will probably not tell the doctor outright. The doctor might even get the impression of a passive-aggressive person who does not behave compliantly. Often, therapies are prematurely terminated and the patient begins "doctor shopping."

Latin America

Medical doctor–patient interactive practices in the Latin American continent are heavily marked by a strong oral tradition rooted in the native indigenous inhabitants' oral culture. This creates a high expectation and demand on the oral interaction in any profession. Thus, high empathy level is expected from the doctor; for example, it would be considered rude if the heath professional is too objective, direct, or abrupt in the announcement of certain illnesses. Among the poorer, less-educated individuals the doctor is still taken as somebody of unquestionable higher knowledge, he/she is considered somehow empowered with a certain superior capability to sort out any kind of physical or mental health problem; here prevails the belief that what the doctor says is "right" (Garrafa and Albuquerque 2001).

The Private and the Public Health-Care System Doctor–patient relationships are also affected by the type of health-care system. There are mainly two outstanding types: the private and the public one. Public health care means free medical care for all. This overloads the public system and promotes serious deficiency of quality in the public sector, which is promoting a rapid expansion in the private sector, already reaching 25 % of the population in Brazil, for example. Evidence shows both systems are putting doctors and other personal under stress with time constraints and low salaries, which is promoting more and more cuts in the time doctors spend with each patient. Consequently, this brings a reasonable amount of dissatisfaction affecting significantly interaction quality between doctor–patient in a culture that relies mostly on orally oriented practices.

New Media Patients' easy access to information is allowing more and more patients to come to the doctor with almost ready self-established diagnoses of what he/she believes the supposed health "problem" is, and more than that, also with a made-up mind of what he/she believes must take as medication. This, at times, has proven to be strenuous in cases where there is no real need of prescribed medication or where the diagnosis is very different from the one brought by the patient.

Africa

The Paternalistic Model In Uganda, there are barriers that may restrict the clinician to just one model—the paternalistic model. The dominant health-care system in Uganda is the Western or modern health care; the Western-trained doctor has the Western views of health and disease while the patient has cultural views or beliefs about health and disease. Any model that gives powers to the patient is undermined when the patient and the doctor have different views or beliefs about the problem, and yet the dominant health-care system favors the views/beliefs of the Western-trained doctor.

There is low health literacy and generally low education. This puts the doctor in such a high and powerful position as compared to the patient who may be poor, have low education and a poor social status. The doctor is therefore seen as "all knowing." Any attempts to try and devolve power to the patient is met by remarks such as "Dr., you are the one who knows." The situation of a heavy burden of communicable diseases such as HIV, malaria and other parasitic diseases, pneumonia, diarrhea, tuberculosis, coupled with a very limited number of doctors persistently leaves the doctor with no choice but to be paternalistic in the relationship with the patient.

In a collective society, there is a lack of individuality in psychological functioning, a lesser focus on individualized human rights and the associated tendency toward overriding patient autonomy, as, for example, a wife will at best wait for her husband to make decisions that affect her own health; otherwise even the whole clan could have a say.

References

Balint M. The doctor, his patient and the illness. 2nd. edn. London: Pitman: 1964. 3rd Millenium edition, 2000. Edinburgh: Churchill Livingstone; 2000.

Garaffa V, Albuquerque MC. Enfoque bioético de la comunicación en la relación médico-paciente em las unidades de terapia intensiva pediátrica. Acta Bioeth. 2001;7(2):355–67.

Nilchaikovit T, Hill JM, Holland JC. The effects of culture on illness behavior and medical care: Asian and American differences. Gen HospPsychiat. 1993;15:41–50.

Chapter 6
Doctor–Patient Communication

Kurt Fritzsche, Axel Schweickhardt, Gertrud Frahm, Sonia Diaz Monsalve, Hamid Afshar Zanjani, Farzad Goli

A patient's cooperation and thus the success or failure of medical treatment depends on the quality of the doctor–patient communication. The most important diagnostic and therapeutic act of a doctor is the medical interview. A doctor conducts up to 200,000 interviews with patients and their families in the course of his career. In most specialties, one-third of the doctor's time is taken up with interviews. Seventy percent of all diagnoses can be made based on the anamnesis interview.

K. Fritzsche (✉) · S. D. Monsalve
Department of Psychosomatic Medicine and Psychotherapy,
University Medical Center, Hauptstr. 8, 79104 Freiburg, Germany
e-mail: kurt.fritzsche@uniklinik-freiburg.de

S. D. Monsalve
e-mail: sonia.diaz-monsalve@uniklinik-freiburg.de

A. Schweickhardt
Potenziale GmbH Business Consultants,
Peyerstr. 34, 90429 Nuremberg, Germany
e-mail: Schweickhardt@potenziale.biz

G. Frahm
Department of Human Sciences, Federal University of Paraná,
R. Gal. Carneiro, 460, Curitiba, PR 80060-150, Brazil
e-mail: gfrahm@uol.com.br

H. Afshar Zanjani
Department of Psychiatry, Isfahan University of Medical Sciences, Isfahan, Iran
e-mail: afshar@med.mui.ac.ir; shafsharz@gmail.com

Noor Hospital, Isfahan, Iran

F. Goli
Department of bioenergy economy,
Energy Medicine University, California, USA
e-mail: Dr.fgoli@yahoo.com

Danesh-e Tandorosti Institute, Isfahan, Iran
e-mail: info@iranianhealth.com

K. Fritzsche et al. (eds.), *Psychosomatic Medicine,* DOI 10.1007/978-1-4614-1022-5_6,

Table 6.1 Patient-centered interview

Transferring patient-centered interview
Let the patient finish talking
Use open-ended questions
Pause
Encourage the patient to continue talking
Paraphrase
Summarize the contents
Reflect the patient's emotions

In the first part of this chapter, the basics of a patient-centered and doctor-centered interview are presented. In the second part, the application of these interview techniques will be presented using the example of biopsychosocial history and dealing with aggressive and demanding patients.

Patient-centered interview

Active listening is the most important method in patient-centered interviews. The doctor plays the role of the listener, but is definitely not passive. He concentrates on the question of what contents are relevant for the patient. The doctor is also active, since he makes it clear to the patient with listener signals ("mhm," "yes") and postures that he is following his presentation. This style is recommended in the first part of the interview and especially in emotional situations, or if the patient himself talks about psychosocial stress.

Table 6.1 lists the techniques of patient-centered interviews, which will be explained in more detail below.

Let the Patient Finish Talking, Give Him Space

Studies show that doctors already interrupt patients for the first time after 15–20 s. Usually an open-ended first question (like: "What brings you here today?") signals to the patient that he has space to speak. If the doctor lets the patient finish what he is saying, then it has been found that patients are more cooperative, keep their comments short, and only talk about relevant things. The average patient speaking time at the beginning of an interview is 92 s, and 78 % of patients stop within 2 min (Langewitz et al. 2002).

Open-Ended Questions

Open-ended questions are those that cannot be answered with a simple yes or no. By using open-ended questions, the doctor allows the patient space and signals that he is interested in the patient's point of view. If, however, the patient cannot find the right words, it can be meaningful to help him with closed questions. No additional questions or explanations should be added after an open question has been asked, since the question will then curtain its supportive, patient-centered function.

Pause

A short pause of about 3 s has been found to be effective. In short pauses of silence, ideas occur to the patient that they may have forgotten. The pause permits the patient to continue speaking if there is something to add. The patient may express thoughts he/she had hesitated to address. The pause lowers the inhibition threshold for speaking about psychosocial matters. During the pause, the doctor emphasizes by listener signals ("hmm," "yes") and by his posture that he is listening to the patient and wants to give him the opportunity to continue speaking. Contrary to the fear that pauses might be interpreted as incompetence, pauses act as relief. It is pleasant to be able to think about something briefly. The doctor appears interested, calm, and sure.

Case Study "Pause"
Doctor: You mentioned briefly stress at work; can you tell me more about that?
Patient: Hmm, yes. The problem is that the company is not in a very solid position. And now there was a large recall action that had to be dealt with quickly to prevent further damage. That meant we all had to work overtime; that takes a lot out of you.
Doctor: Hmm... (3 s pause)
Patient: ... to be honest, I just can't go on. I have trouble dragging myself out of bed in the morning and trouble falling asleep at night. And there are often arguments with my wife. And I can't blame her. When I come home at night, I'm often irritable and haven't energy to do much of anything. Actually, I could do with a week's vacation, but that's impossible at the moment.

Encourage the Patient to Continue Talking

Nonverbal signs like nodding when the patient hesitates encourages him indirectly to continue speaking. Eye contact signals attention and interest, and also encourages patients to continue speaking. Posture facing the patient emphasizes the doctor's presence. Verbal possibilities to encourage the patient to speak are short expressions like "mhm" or "ah yes."

Paraphrase

Paraphrasing means repeating what has been said by the patient in one's own words. The doctor takes on the patient's viewpoint and focuses on that part of what the patient said that has the greatest relevant content. Using paraphrases is a good way to support the patient in emotional or personal topics. Questions tend more to disrupt. Paraphrasing often brings new perspectives for the patient that lead to what can be astounding solutions.

Case Study "Paraphrase"
Patient: Couldn't we postpone the next chemotherapy cycle?
Doctor: You would like to have a longer pause?
Patient: Yes. You see, it's like this: My sister lives in the USA and is coming for a visit in 2 weeks. I can't visit her at the moment, and the medications make me so tired. Well, it would be really dumb while she is here.
Doctor: Ah yes, you don't want to be hampered while your sister is here?
Patient: Yes, that's it. Actually, I don't want her to realize so much that I'm sick. I mean, she knows it, of course, but she shouldn't have to be confronted with it.
Doctor: Mhm, you don't want your sister to see you as sick.
Patient: Yes, I don't want pity or so from her. You see, I'm the older one and I was always there when she needed me.
Doctor: OK, I understand. You don't want pity and help from your little sister.
Patient: Well, if she helps a little that's OK, but no pity.

While the first paraphrase focuses on the treatment, the doctor addresses the stress and the patient's personal background in the later ones. This reflects the background of the patient's rejection for her. Often, the patients themselves will then arrive at a new solution. If this is not the case, the doctor can help.
Doctor: Could you imagine telling her that you don't want pity?
Patient: Actually, it's silly. I'm still strong enough to deal with my sister's sympathy and I can tell her that I don't want her to pity me.

Summarize the Contents

With paraphrasing, the doctor only picks up on the most important parts of the message, whereas summarizing covers a larger segment of the discussion. The doctor says in his own words what he has understood. The patient can then add information he had forgotten. This leads to agreement between the doctor and the patient. The doctor checks whether he has understood what the patient said. Summaries are also a suitable means of transition to a new discussion or to announce the end by summarizing the most important contents. In this way, it is also a doctor-centered communication technique.

Table 6.2 Doctor-centered interview

Taking over the doctor-centered interview
Transparency
Of contents
Of the environment
Of the interview phases
Doctor-centered question types
Interrupting
Metacommunicative comments

Reflect the Patient's Emotions

Reflecting emotions is very similar to paraphrasing. However, the reflection refers primarily to emotional contents. Sometimes, these emotions are addressed directly. Sometimes, the response to emotions is based on an observation of body reaction or refers to what is said between the lines.

Case Study "Reflecting emotions"
Patient: I'm afraid it could be a malignant tumor.
Doctor: You are anxious and worried about what the examination will reveal.
Patient: My mother had a fatal accident 3 weeks ago. (Cries)
Doctor: You become very sad when you think of that event.

The doctor then waits to see whether the patient permits the doctor to pick up on his emotion. In the pause, he can collect his own feelings. Once the doctor has described the feeling, the patient has the possibility of talking further or changing the subject.

After an intensive emotional statement, it is especially important that the doctor pauses and does not immediately soothe or change the subject. For the patient, it is important that he does not feel dismissed but rather gains the doctor's interest and sympathy. He experiences that emotions are acceptable.

Pitfalls

- A common mistake is to give too much advice. In terms of partner relationships, advice is reasonable when it comes to medical expertise, but less appropriate the more psychosocial concerns are associated with the advice.

Doctor-centered interview

A doctor-centered interview includes many structuring techniques (Table 6.2). They help to focus and streamline the interview. Thus, they complement the already-discussed patient-centered interviewing techniques.

Table 6.3 Transparency

Transparency of content
Provide information about the treatment steps that you have planned for this appointment
Provide the necessary technical information
Inform the patient why you do, what you do
Transparency of the environment
Point out potential trouble
Provide information about the timing of the interview
Transparency of the interview phases
Make it clear if you expect from your patient longer explanations or short answers
Indicate transitions between patient-centered and doctor-centered interview
Announce the conclusion of the interview well in advance

Transparency

The basic instrument for keeping within time limits is the transparency of the interview contents, the timeframe, and the transitions between various interview phases. The transition to a new interview phase should be clearly emphasized. Table 6.3 lists important techniques for providing transparency.

Questions in a Doctor-Centered Interview

Table 6.4 lists the question types that serve to structure a doctor-centered interview.

Case Study "Counter questions"
Doctor: In my opinion, general anesthesia is suitable for your child because she is too young to remain calm with a local anesthetic.
Patient (Slightly aggressive): Would you do the same to your own child?
Doctor: I'll answer your question in a moment; first, can you tell me beforehand what's behind your question? (*Counter question*)
Patient: I would like to know if the risk is really justifiable, you see. If you are not personally affected, such decisions may be too simple.
Doctor: I have children of my own and would do the same for them also. But it is more important to me, what risk you can justify yourself? (*Alternating the level of discussion*)

Table 6.4 Question types to structure a doctor-centered interview

Closed-ended questions	Questions that can be answered with yes, no, or a short statement Allow to query specific information "Are you vaccinated against tetanus?"
Alternative questions	Already provide different answers "Is the discharge green, brown, or yellowish?"
Knowledge questions	A doctor can provide more targeted information when he queries the knowledge of the patient in advance "Have you yourself looked for information about how one can cure your pain?"
Opinion questions	Target value systems Problems can be anticipated, priorities regarding the course may be set "How do you feel about taking medication?"
Counter questions	In case of patient questions with unclear intention More information before answer Often particularly useful in case of aggressive, difficult patients
Leading questions	The interviewee is given a specific answer "You certainly also don't want to feel any pain?" Overall these questions should be avoided, only if it is considered to be appropriate after careful weighing, trying to convince a patient
Behavioral questions	Express the request to do something specific "Can you summarize this in your own words once again?"

Interrupting

Over the course of the interview, it may be necessary to stop the flow of speech of some patients in order to stay on topic. Interrupting is usually perceived as impolite, and must be done in a way so that the patient can accept it and returns to the topic.

The Four Elements of Interruption

- *Direct interruption*
  The doctor addresses the patient by name, looks him in the eye, and might even touch his arm.
- *Summarizing*
  The doctor signals that he has understood that the topic is important to the patient, even if the discussion cannot be continued at present.
- *Repeat interview goal*
  The doctor repeats the goal of the interview, even the consequence if the structure is not maintained.
- *Obtain agreement*
  At the end, the doctor asks if the patient agrees to the procedure. This makes it possible for him to remind the patient of the agreement if other interruptions occur.

Metacommunication Comments

Metacommunication comments are comments about the way the interview is being conducted. They can help to structure an interview.

Case Study "Metacommunication comments"
Doctor: It occurs to me that we very quickly digress from the subject of an operation, although I had expected it would be at the center of our conversation.
Patient: Well, yes, it's true. I'm also pretty nervous just thinking about it.
Doctor: Shall we postpone the interview?
Patient: No, at some point we have to discuss it.

Pitfalls

- Several questions are asked one after the other.
- The transitions from one topic to the next are not clear.
- The interruption occurs too late, the anger at the patient becomes apparent.
- Metacommunication comments are phrased as allegations rather than observations.

Depending on the situation and the patient's personality, the interview style may be more patient centered or more doctor centered. In a medical emergency, the doctor must obtain an overview of the situation and make a tentative diagnosis by asking the patient or accompanying relative specific short questions: "Are you in pain? Are you a diabetic? What medications do you take?" In emotional crisis situations, the doctor provides the patient with an opportunity for emotional relief, summarizes what he/she heard in his/her own words, and reflects the emotions of the patient. The following two typical interview situations are presented, where both patient-centered and physician-centered interview techniques are necessary in a balanced manner.

Interview situations

The Biopsychosocial Anamnesis

The anamnesis is the most frequent discussion form in the hospital and practice. A different procedure is needed in emergency admissions of a hospital than in the family doctor's office. The phases presented here are based on the case in which the doctor hardly has any previous information about the patient and there is no immediate need for treatment (as for example in acute pain). Depending on the task at hand, the doctor is forced to choose certain phases or to omit them entirely and go back to them later.

Greeting

The greeting gives the impression of how attentive and interested the doctor is in the patient. For the doctor, it is professional routine, but for the patient, the appointment is coupled with a number of hopes and fears. The frequent blood pressure increase in the doctor's office ("white coat hypertension") is witness to this. Some brief *small talk* facilitates the first contact. One or two sentences about the family, the weather, the trip to the office bridge the feeling of strangeness, provide the physician with beginning information in a format that is comfortable for the patient and family. It is also part of the greeting that the doctor briefly introduces himself and his function.

Patient-Centered Phase of the Anamnesis

The patient describes what he wants. With the patient-centered interview, the doctor supports this presentation. He should not interrupt in this phase, unless something is unclear. In this phase, the doctor receives information about the complaints, the patient's life situation, and quality of life, and how this has changed due to the illness. Finally, the doctor can learn something about the patient's personal understanding of how the disease came about and is maintained, and about the resources available to the patient to cope with the disease.

Case Study "Patient-centered anamnesis"
Doctor: You have just indicated that it's not easy for your children to deal with your illness. I'd be interested to know more about it.

The patient may be irritated, since it has been his experience that doctors block such topics. He may react as follows:
Patient: I don't know. There's nothing I can do about it anyway.

The doctor can then explain why he thinks it's relevant and leave it to the patient whether he wishes to speak about it further.
Doctor: I don't know if we can change anything there. But it's important for me that you have as little stress during treatment as possible. If you want to, you can tell me more.

Psychosocial Anamnesis

In an initially somatic-directed anamnesis, data about the life history, such as serious illnesses or hospitalizations in childhood, or stress from the illness or death of a parent, may be expressed. This information enables the doctor to form first hypotheses about a relationship between early stress and the current complaints:

- Psychosocial topics
- Individual anamnesis
- Family
- Family environment: parenting style of the parents, emotional climate, relationship between the parents, relationship among siblings, etc.
- Diseases, disease risks, disease management, and health behavior in the family
- Early childhood development: specific diseases, hospitalizations, etc.
- Typical threshold situations like school years, puberty, moving out of the parents' home, choice of profession, marriage, retirement, etc.
- Current life situation, for example job, family changes in occupational and professional life
- Forms of coping with disease, such as active or depressive coping, denial of the severity of the symptoms
- Subjective understanding of the cause of disease

Doctor-Centered Phase of the Anamnesis

In the doctor-centered phase of the anamnesis, the doctor asks specific closed questions in order to obtain as quickly as possible the information he needs to make the diagnosis. The often-used history sheets help to ask all the questions necessary and signals the altered interview style to the patient.

Physical Examination

Even in the physical examination, there are verbal and nonverbal exchange processes between the doctor and the patient. Touching during the physical examination can be experienced as an advance by a stranger that violates bodily limits, is intimate and/or penetrating. For example, in examination of the abdomen, the degree of needed tension depends on the examiner's sensitivity and the trust the patient has in the situation. The patient may experience feelings of resistance, fear, shame, or pain.

> **Practical Tip** The *perception* and *feedback* of physical reactions to the patient may help the patient to relax, gain trust, and feel that the doctor understands him.
>
> "I notice that you are tensing your stomach. Is being touched unpleasant?"

Treatment Planning

The goal of treatment planning is to find with the patient a treatment strategy that combines the patient's willingness with medical necessity to the greatest extent possible (*shared decision making*). What we know of compliance is sobering. In family practice, only 33 % of the patients take their medications correctly. So, it is highly relevant whether the patient can or will follow the treatment at all.

Conclusion

The concluding phase serves as a review. The doctor again summarizes, bringing together the topics that were discussed and the most important points. Here, the patient has the chance to add anything important. The doctor then decides whether the additions should be clarified immediately or at a later date.

Pitfalls

- Switching between patient-centered and physician-centered approach is not announced. This can irritate and confuse the patient, because he cannot understand the interview structure.
- The doctor does not end the interview in time. Right before the conclusion of the interview the patient brings up another important topic for discussion. The doctor addresses it and exceeds the time frame.

Interviews with Challenging and Aggressive Patients—the CALM Model

Case Study "Mr. G"

Mr. G. is questioned in the doctor's office of the cardiology department. He is facing junior doctor Dr. B. Puzzled, Mr. G. pauses, looking questioningly at Dr. B., then around the room, then back at Dr. B. Dr. B. asks Mr. G. to take a seat. In response, there is only a clearly impatient and rude question: "Where is Prof. K.? I had an appointment with her." Quickly and apologetically, Dr. B. answers, "Prof. K. is attending an international conference at which she was invited to give the opening speech." Dr. B. cannot finish the last sentence, because Mr. G. bursts out, and with a reproachful, loud voice he complains, insults the clinic, the lack of organization, and, eventually, Dr. B. who becomes smaller and smaller.

The CALM model is a graduated model used to de-escalate conflict-prone discussions. Generally, the stages should be run through in ascending order. The two

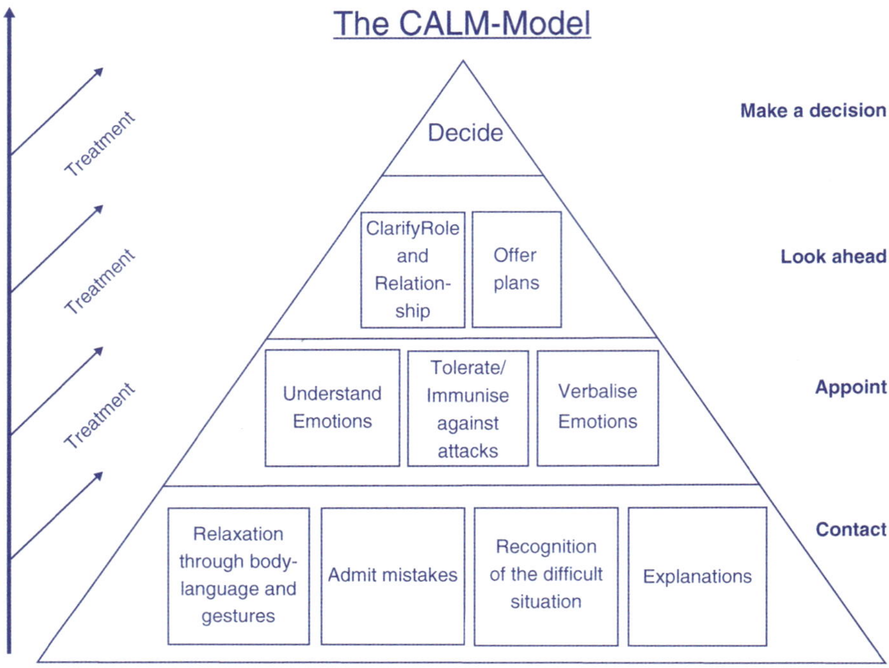

Fig. 6.1 The CALM model

lower stages conserve or strengthen the relationship, while the two top stages are agreements that constitute a compromise in the form of a last common denominator between the clinician and the patient. If the stages are implemented skillfully, the top of the pyramid is only reached in rare cases (Fig. 6.1).

Stage 1: Contact

The purpose of Stage 1 is to maintain contact with the patient in spite of his/her aggressive or degrading behavior. In so doing, it is essential to keep the aggressions at bay and to remain calm and objective. Initial aggression should be allowed to surge and ebb away like a wave, and it should under no circumstances be suppressed. It may be helpful to accept the fact that the patient is in a difficult situation or else he/she would not behave in such an inappropriate way. They may launch bitter accusations at you, but the initial focus should be on the patient's situation, and no excuses should be made. The body language is particularly important to allow the aggression to surge. It should be emphasized that the patient's concerns are understood and will be considered. These procedures are usually sufficient to appease the situation. Should this not be the case, follow up with Stage 2.

Case Study "Contact"
Patient: That really is the limit. I have a serious heart condition and drive 200 km to get to this clinic, and then you tell me that everything is in vain? Last time, everything was urgent, and now we are canceling the appointment just like that? To the first doctor that comes along, do you think because of you I'm driving this far? Are you even a doctor?
Doctor (Quiet and approachable): Mr. G., I'm very sorry, I thought you had been informed that Prof. K. is out of town. Let's have a seat.
Patient (A little calmer): Hmm (Louder again), here, does one hand know what the other does?
Doctor: Please have a seat; then, I would like to explain everything, as far as I can.
Patient (Breathes and then sits down): But don't think that this matter can be resolved easily.

Stage 2: Appoint

The purpose of the second phase is to name the observed emotion directly. The anger, the frustration, the disappointment are addressed directly. Often, directly addressing the emotion causes a temporary aggravation of the latter. However, you should be aware of this and "ignore it." The level of the emotionality will then quickly drop considerably. This is the time when it comes to focusing on the patient's self-revelation within the scope of the four-ears model (see Chap. 1) and to address the emotions responsible for the aggressive behavior. Raw emotions are usually the result of fears or worries. If the latter are addressed, the quality of the discussion can rapidly change.

In rare cases, patients refuse to cooperate on this level. If this happens, you will have to move to Stage 3 and look for the common denominator to carry on the collaboration.

Case Study "Appoint"
Patient: You think you'll get away that easily? You are absolutely wrong. I have many influential friends and contacts with hospital management. I'll let them know what's going on here.
Doctor: I understand that you are very outraged.
Patient: Outraged, yes, you can say that. I am outraged, yes.
Doctor: Hmm... (Brief pause)
Patient (A bit calmer): I have every reason to be. This is about my health, perhaps, even about my life, and I simply expect the best treatment. Do you think otherwise I would come here?

Doctor: There is also a lot of fear. I wonder what should happen next.
Patient (Now thoughtfully): Yes, that's no easy task when it comes to the heart. You see, I have confidence in Prof. K. because I know I am in good hands.
Doctor: That is what this is about, that you feel safe with her.
Patient: Yes, at least I felt this way. Prior to this incident.
Doctor: Yes, confidence is shattered for now.

Stage 3: Look Ahead

The next stage is designed to emphasize the professional relationship between the clinician and the patient. This stage is about clarifying how the collaboration should proceed. The key in this phase is to make the patient aware of the common goal and to make him/her an offer that will be upheld, irrespective of his/her frustration. The limits are specified and the rules of the game established for the collaboration. It is essential that this is done without resentment.

Case Study "Look ahead"
Doctor: I realize how angry you are still. For me, the question is now, how we proceed from here.
Patient: Proceeding. Proceeding, how. . . ?
Doctor (Interrupts): I would like to point out once again that Prof. K. has told me all findings, that I am well prepared for the interview with you, and that I would like to walk you through the findings. At the next appointment with Prof. K. you can discuss the operation before deciding for a treatment option. Thus, your trip would not be in vain, and you could still discuss all relevant steps with Prof. K. I would be glad if this approach could resolve this issue at least to a small extent.

Stage 4: Make a Decision

During this phase, the patient will be presented with a "contract" he/she may or may not sign. Consequently, the patient is put in charge of his/her further treatment and he/she will have to make his/her own decision. Reaching this stage means that the escalation has progressed to an advanced stage. Therefore, it may be helpful to offer the patient time for reflection, by taking a walk or by sleeping over the decision.

Case Study "Make a decision"
Doctor: Mr. G., I think any more discussion won't get us anywhere. I would like to offer to let you know the findings, but you must decide whether you

would like this or not.
Patient: What do you mean by deciding? How should I decide? I don't even know you.
Doctor: I think I've told you all I can say. If you need some more time, then you may take a seat in the waiting room or take a walk. When you come back, I'll see you as quickly as possible.
Patient: Okay, a walk might be a good idea, but better not make me wait for long.
Doctor: Please see the receptionist; I'll let them know to notify me immediately.

Pitfalls

- The doctor fails to distance himself/herself from his/her own troubles. While being superficially friendly, a hidden sharp tongue is apparent in his/her comments. This is enough to complicate the interview even more. It is therefore important that one's anger is actually overcome.
- The switch to level 3 is too fast without having recognized or resolved the issues of the emotional level sufficiently. This increases the likelihood of discontinuation of treatment on the part of the patient.

Practical Tip There are situations in which the angry patient speaks what he may feel and the doctor quickly is pushed into the role of the just attacked. In such situations, the following steps are helpful:

- Ask the patient in a friendly but determined way to come into the doctor's office.
- Offer him/her a chair—sitting makes aggression more difficult.
- In no case hide out behind books or your desk; an open attitude is more likely to calm him/her down.
- Maintain a proper distance: too close can be provocative or threatening, too far away may be understood as an attempt at evasion or inaccessibility.

Cultural Aspects

General

The manner in which patients present their symptoms initially depends largely on their cultural background and the associated patterns and norms as to how to talk about diseases and mental health issues in general. In many cultures, emotional issues and personal feelings are considered a personal matter, talking about them is equivalent to publicly exposing oneself. Even family conflicts are widely regarded as internal matters which are not communicated externally. To ask for sexual habits and difficulties represents a particularly large hurdle for doctors. In Asian countries, the anatomical terms "penis" and "vagina" are largely avoided and replaced with coded phrases. Even the sexual act is described with different expressions and disguises depending on the culture. Male impotency is a taboo issue mostly with less educated patients. Patients tend to avoid addressing the problem directly. In these cases, doctors have to be very skilled to address such culturally delicate matters.

Other taboos include death and dying. For example, in Micronesia asking about the reason for the death of parents involves the fear of punishment. It is also important not to discuss mistakes and omissions of the parents in front of children, because this could hurt the image of parents as authority figures.

Also, questions about the financial situation, costs of certain purchases, or even age can hurt the person being questioned.

Latin America

A survey and ethnographic study on doctor–patient interactions, developed by the University of Sao Paulo Medical School, evidenced that doctors still rely mostly on oral orientations (only the prescription of medicine is written), regardless if it relates to a first visit of the patient or not. The study identified two main modes of doctor–patient interactions; in one mode, doctors spend some of the time talking about trivial matters with the patient within a frame of the doctor's friendly attitude, which in the survey has also shown a high score of satisfaction by the patient. In the other mode, doctors adopt more objective procedures of interaction with exclusive concentration on physical examinations and history, strictly focused on the problem presented by the patient; this mode has also evidenced high satisfaction by patients. As regards to the communication skills used by the doctors, the study observed that doctors have been careful in making themselves understood to the patient, using an adequate language in the explanation of more specific medical issues such as exams' interpretations, also making use of colloquial language with less educated patients. As for the time spent with the patient, it is as low as 4 min with each patient (Kiyohara et al. 2001).

The cultural trend of lack of assertiveness in general habitual everyday communication tends to make doctors take a more paternalistic attitude by adopting smaller steps in the communication of certain illnesses; depending on the case, the doctor even opts to talk to the nearest relative(s) or guardian first. It even creates certain *tabus* mostly in the more primitive cultures, which can be traced back to the original native inhabitants' beliefs that certain illnesses have a kind of "sacred aura" that must be preserved and/or taken into account; thus, at times, instead of saying the name of the illness, there is abundant use of paraphrasing. Studies have evidenced the relevance of the bond established between doctor and patient and relatives for the effectiveness of doctors' work; for this empathy demands are crucial, for which some themes related to doctor–patient relationship were pointed out as follows: use of adequate communicating skills, establishment of adequate bond between doctor and patient, adequate therapeutic approach, family inclusion in the interaction, consideration to the suffering status, and the differences in communication abilities (Silva et al. 2011).

Iran

In "Qābus nameh," one of the major Persian literature works of eleventh century, a competent physician is described as follows:

"A doctor should be tenderhearted, wise minded, and good intuition. . . " (Onsor-almali et al. 2006). It means that empathy, logical thinking, and transpersonal cognition are supposed to be the main characteristics of an authentic physician. It could be also inspiring for our contemporary medicine for fostering cognitive, emotional, spiritual, and metacognitive abilities of medical doctors in order to elaborate doctor–patient communication, clinical reasoning, and clinical ethics.

References

Kiyohara LY, Kayano LK, Kobayashi MLT, Alessi MS, Yamamoto MU, Yunes-Filho PRM, et al. The patient-physician interactions as seen by undergraduate medical students. Sao Paulo Med J. 2001; 119(3):97–100.

Langewitz W, Denz M, Keller A, Kiss A, Rüttimann S, Wössmer B. Spontaneous talking time at start of consultation in outpatient clinic: cohort study. BMJ 2002; 325:682–3.

Onsor- Almali KV, Nameh Q, Yusefi GH, Editor. Elmi Farhangi Inc, Tehran; 2006, ch 14, p. 180.

Silva C, Rodrigues C, Lima J, Jucá N, Augusto K, Lino C, et al. Relação médico-paciente em oncologia: medos, angústias e habilidades comunicacionais de médicos na cidade de Fortaleza (CE). Ciênc Saúde Coletiva [online]. 2011; 16(1):1457–65.

Chapter 7
Family Medicine

Werner Geigges, Kurt Fritzsche, Susan H. McDaniel, Xudong Zhao, Catherine Abbo, Gertrud Frahm and Sonia Diaz Monsalve

Case Study "Family A"
Mrs. A., 33 years old, married to Mr. A., 36 years old, mother of a daughter (age 9) and a son (age 11). She is diagnosed with Hodgkin's disease, stage CS IV. At the beginning of the illness, the family stuck together closely: The husband canceled all leisure activities, was very committed to the children, and visited his wife regularly during hospital stays. Complementary relationships were evident: When Mrs. A. showed signs of weakness, her husband demonstrated strength by assuming the role of a primary caregiver and filling in. The children also responded to the mother with a decidedly upbeat attitude, providing her with cheerful children's drawings. Conflicts were played down and harmony and stability were stressed. Ten months after the initial diagnosis of cancer, the family pattern was changing: The 11-year-old son was becoming increasingly aggressive and experienced a drop in school performance. The doctor invited the family to a family interview.

(Continued)

K. Fritzsche (✉) · S. D. Monsalve
Department of Psychosomatic Medicine and Psychotherapy,
University Medical Center, Hauptstr. 8, 79104 Freiburg, Germany
e-mail: kurt.fritzsche@uniklinik-freiburg.de

S. D. Monsalve
e-mail: sonia.diaz-monsalve@uniklinik-freiburg.de

W. Geigges
Rehaklinik Glotterbad,
Gehrenstr. 10, 79286 Glottertal, Germany
e-mail: w.geigges@rehaklinik-glotterbad.de

S. H. McDaniel
Department of Psychiatry, Department of Family Medicine,
University of Rochester Medical Center, 777 S. Clinton Ave, Rochester, NY 14620, USA
e-mail: susanh2_mcdaniel@urmc.rochester.edu

K. Fritzsche et al. (eds.), *Psychosomatic Medicine,* DOI 10.1007/978-1-4614-1022-5_7,

Definition

"We define family as any group of people related either biologically, emotionally, or legally, i.e., the group of people that the patient defines as significant for his/her well-being. The family-oriented practitioner gathers information about these family relationships, patterns of health and illness across generations, emotional connections with deceased and geographically removed members, and life-cycle transitions, in order to understand the patient within his/her larger context. In other words, the family-oriented clinician mobilizes the patient's natural support system to enhance health and well-being" (McDaniel et al. 2005, p. 2).

Relevance

Relatives of a patient will significantly influence the health and illness behavior of the patient and his/her interaction with the doctor and the health care system. Therefore, the family perspective is an important aspect in the context of a biopsychosocial understanding of disease.

Theoretical background

The Concept of the Life Cycle

The concept of the life cycle (Carter and McGoldrick 1989) assumes that families throughout their lives go through different phases such as pairing, parenting, aging, etc. Each of these phases represents a potential threat to the existing organizational structure of the family. A successful completion of the phases is vital for growth and development in families. The phases that families go through can be divided into stages, having characteristic manifestations with signature issues. It is always helpful to consider the developmental stage of the family at the time of the occurrence of disease in a family member.

X. Zhao
Department of Psychosomatic Medicine, Shanghai East Hospital,
Tongji University, 150 Jimo Road, Pudong New Area, 200120 Shanghai, China
e-mail: zhaoxd@tongji.edu.cn

C. Abbo
Department of Psychiatry, Makerere University College of Health Sciences
and Mulago National Referral and Teaching Hospital, Mulago Hill Road,
7072 Kampala, Uganda
e-mail: cathyabbo@chs.mak.ac.ug, cathya180@gmail.com

G. Frahm
Department of Human Sciences, Federal University of Paraná,
R. Gal. Carneiro, 460, Curitiba, PR 80060-150, Brazil
e-mail: gfrahm@uol.com.br

The Young Couple

The relationship of a young couple, which is in the process of replacing the family of origin and building a new family system, is often threatened if one partner becomes seriously ill. The affected person can fall back into the dependence and intimacy of his/her family of origin, who may take care of upcoming decisions without including the partner adequately.

Families with Adolescent Children

The main task of this phase of development is the gradual but definite separation of the children who turn more and more to the peer group and are looking for their own identity and their own life goals. In such a situation, a serious illness of a family member can easily lead to termination or suspension of this separation dynamics. Regression trends and dependency-autonomy conflicts can result. Individuation efforts are often associated with guilt, called the separation guilt.

At Old Age

In the later phase of aging, the spirit of partnership among parents and interaction with their adult children depends largely on how the phase of adolescence and its troubles have been managed. Being separate with a simultaneous feeling of togetherness is very important for this phase of older adulthood. In working with seriously ill elderly patients, the relationship with their grandchildren is often seen as one of the key coping resources, closely linked with the feeling of "still being needed."

Family as a Resource and Support System

Family-based interventions, such as a change in eating habits or to reduce cardiopulmonary risk factors, are more successful and cost-effective than programs that focus only on the individual patient. Spouses or significant others have greater influence on health-related habits than any other person, including the attending doctor.

In case of severe disease, the partners and family can play a positive support role through the following:

- Experience of being accepted despite the disease
- Experience of being able to provide something to their spouse despite a serious illness
- New common ground through dialogue and joint activities
- New emotional closeness
- Allowing feelings of grief and love

Family as a Burdened System

The transition from acute to chronic disease with the need to provide for chronically ill patients both at home and in the hospital, places increasing burden on families. In addition to mental diseases, severe physical diseases of a parent play a role in the relationship between parent and child in many ways and can result in lasting damage to the psychosocial development. Particularly in cancer and neurological diseases, maladaptive coping patterns can be found in up to 50 % of the children. In the case of a disease, the following stressors can occur in families and partnerships:

- A shift of the balance between give and take, and change of the distribution of tasks within the partnership
- Unresolved chronic conflicts that no longer can be avoided or suppressed under the burden of the physical disease
- Feelings of alienation through physical and mental overload of both partners, and due to behavioral and personality changes in the patient
- Increased helplessness, aggression, feelings of disgust, and associated guilt in the patient and/or caregiver

In the collaboration with patients and their families within health care, we consider families both as a support system and an important resource in managing disease and as system burdened by diseases.

Practical Implementation

The Genogram

The routine use of disease-related genograms proved to be a simple and straightforward technique in the context of family diagnostic and formation of hypotheses. Genograms are graphic representations of a family constellation spanning across multiple generations. It shows in a clear representation positions within the birth order, deaths, diseases, symptoms, life events, etc. They are created as part of a medical history interview with individuals or families (Fig. 7.1).

The proposal to create a genogram can be introduced by the doctor in the following way: "We have talked in detail about your problem. Now I would like to get an overview about the diseases that have occurred in your family. As you tell me about it, I will take notes together with you so that I can recall at a later time who is who." By constructing a family genogram together, there will be numerous opportunities to enter into an in-depth discussion with the patient.

Practical Tip Questions for the genogram

- What diseases run in your family?
- What "counts" as a disease?
- Who is affected?

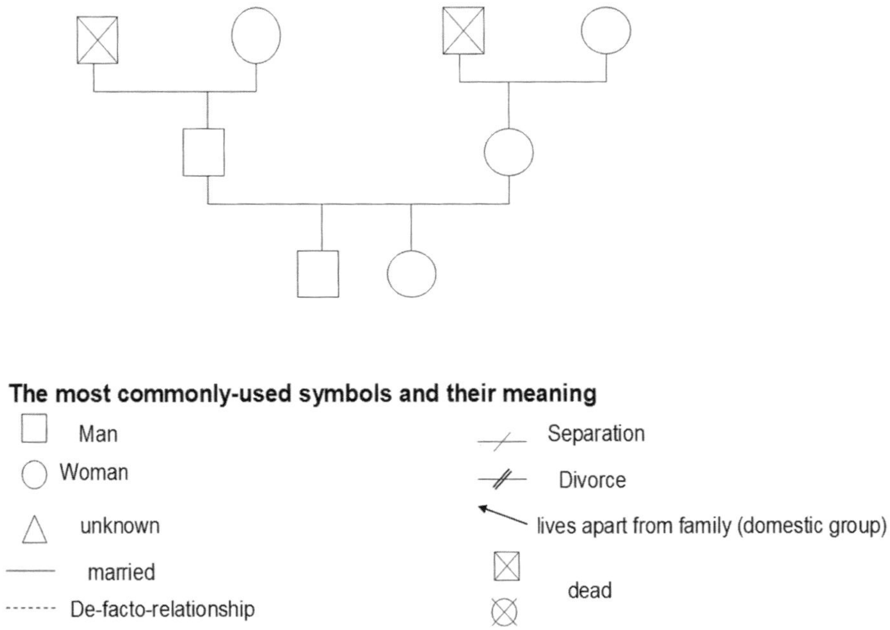

Fig. 7.1 Genogram

- Who cares for the sick?
- What does he/she get for it?
- How did your family deal with illness and death?
- What was the cause of death?
- What coping strategies does your family use for illness, or grieving?

The creation of the genogram takes place in three steps:

1. All members of a family and their relationships are recorded. It is started with the children or the couple as the core family. Then, grandparents are added. Overall, as far as possible, at least three generations should be included.
2. In the second step, information about the family history is added: age, marriage, divorce, miscarriages, death, and serious diseases as well as critical family events.
3. Finally, the quality of relationships among family members may be particularly highlighted.

The Family Dialogue in the Medical Context—Useful Strategies

In the medical context, McDaniel et al. (2005) suggest the therapeutic strategies listed below for couple or family dialogues.

Disease: An Explanation of the Diagnosis, Treatment, Disease Progression, Prognosis

The disease and its impact on the family members, rather than the family conflict as is the case in psychotherapeutic interviews, are at the center of the family dialogue in the medical context. The physician may begin with an explanation of the disease, its prognosis, and the probable course of the disease for the family. Then psychological and social interactions are related to the medical problems.

Inquiring About Medical History

If, as part of a family dialogue, we—the doctors—listen to the medical history of the patient and understand it, we enter the world of the patient and his/her family. In addition to the content of these stories, this approach builds trust for joint work with the family. Important questions in a family dialogue include:

- How does the family cope with and overcome life events and life crises?
- Are there typical patterns within the family on how to deal with illness?
- Is there support across generations in dealing with the illness of a family member?
- What are the constructions of reality in terms of etiology, course, and management of disease or successful healing strategies included in these stories?

Focus on Concerns of the Family

When dealing with a family coping with the stress of a serious illness, it is important not to criticize from the outset or disqualify their coping patterns even, when viewed from the outside, they appear to be rather dysfunctional. Instead, acknowledge their attempts to cope with the current situation and the contribution of individuals to maintain the continued functioning of the whole family. This approach serves to reduce blame and guilt and causes an immediate emotional relief.

Promotion of an Open Communication Between the Parties

Give the family time to process information about prognosis, disease progression, and the treatment plan. Offering the opportunity to continue the dialogue, encouraging them to also ask critical questions and express any objections.

It is particularly important to acknowledge that all family members are concerned, and to help them to express any possible feelings of dismay. Emotional reactions often result in strong uncertainty and helplessness among family members. Dealing with directly or indirectly expressed feelings helps the individual persons concerned. Confrontational statements should be avoided.

The Doctor as the Moderator

If the doctor understands his/her role in the family dialogue to be the moderator, without giving advice, an open exchange within the family can be encouraged. The family will feel they are able to promote and support the positive course of therapy for their loved one.

Phases of the Family Dialogue

Phase 1: Joining

Joining means to connect with each family member and to convey, that one cares to get to know his/her opinion. The dialogue starts after the doctor has greeted each one (even the younger family members) with a handshake, asked for the name, and perhaps the age of the individual family members.

> **Case Study (Continued)** "Joining 1"
> Dr.: "Hello. Thank you all for coming today. I have seen you, Mrs. A., now several times and we have spoken about your illness. I thought it might be helpful to talk together with you and your family about the situation and see what impact the disease has on all of you. We can think together about how all of you can best support your mother and each other."
> (Continued)

As a next step, explain the focus of the conversation and how long it may last.

> **Case Study (Continued)** "Joining 2"
> Dr.: "I have known you, Mrs. A., and you, Mr. A., for many years. However, I know your children just barely. Who would like to introduce the family a bit more in detail? Please again give me their names and ages? Maybe each of you can say a few words, about the person sitting next to him/her."
> (Continued)

Phase 2: Context and Task Clarification

- Institutional context: Especially in the clinical context, it is important that the doctor responsible for the diagnostic and therapeutic process is directly involved in the joint family dialogue. Otherwise there is a high risk that the family will have to deal with varying professional perspectives on the disease and its consequences, which can lead to additional burden.

- Mission clarification—different family caretakers: It should be clarified what other doctors, psychotherapists, and other health professionals are involved in the health problems of the whole family, and how these other professionals think about and assess the current crisis of the family.
- Expectations of the family interview.

Case Study (Continued) "Context and mission clarification"

- *"What needs to be discussed today, so that it was worth your while to come here?"*
- *"For whom was it the most difficult to come here?"*
- To Anna and Paul: *"How did your father explain to you why you should come here today?"*
- *"Who in the family was most looking forward to, or skeptical of, the idea of a joint family meeting?"*
- *"Paul, how did your father manage it so that all of you have taken the time today to come here and have a joint meeting?"*

(Continued)

The questions are intended to encourage direct communication within the family. The family interactions thus initiated offer the opportunity to closely observe how people are talking to each other, who supports or disrespects whom, how the family hierarchy presents itself, and who plays what role in the family. It is important that everyone has the opportunity to express his/her needs and expectations as well as fears and anxieties.

Phase 3: The Disease and its Impact—Views from Different Perspectives

Disease

- What has changed in the family since the onset of the illness?
- What has been tried already by the family to help the patient?
- What does the family know about the disease diagnosis?
- What is your understanding of the therapeutic intervention and side effects?
- What is your belief about the prognosis?

Threat to Family Relationships and Future Plans

- How are roles, relationships, and communication patterns defined within the family?
- According to which patterns are decisions made within the family, currently and before the disease?

- What are the objectives and plans of the family, and how does this disease affect them?
- How does each family member view the changes that were triggered by the disease?

Available Resources

- What financial resources are available, for example, if an income is lost?
- What are the resources in the social network of the family: family, friends, support groups, etc.?

Previous Experience with Similar Situations

- What are the coping strategies used by the family in previous crises?
- What is the medical history of the family and what were the associated experiences of the family?

Phase 4: Treatment Planning

By joining, continuous assessment of the health problems and associated relationship realities, an idea about possible change takes shape.

Case Study (continued) "Treatment planning"
Dr.: "What would be a good final result of our family discussion?

Do you have specific ideas about what could be changed, and how it could be accomplished, so that all of you feel better?"

(Continued)

Phase 5: The Conclusion of the Dialogue

Positive assessment: Each person will be acknowledged in a positive and appreciative way in relation to the family and to the presented problem and the performance of the family as a whole. Problematic behaviors should be described in terms of understandable but suboptimal attempts to cope with the situation.

Homework: In the final phase, the meeting and the main conclusions are summarized. The family's positive resources and strengths are emphasized. Unresolved issues and topics are named. Specific tasks are distributed among the family members.

Case Study (Continued) "Homework"
Dr.: "At the moment I am under the impression that the illness is permanently in your living room—how would it be possible to send it for a walk for a few hours?"

The end of the dialogue also includes support and advice, including:

- Information about local support groups for patients and families
- Information on how other families have mastered a serious illness
- Establishing contact with other such families

During a family dialogue, the basic attitude is impartiality. The doctor is guided by the assumption that, in principle, there is a diversity of individually experienced realities in any family. In the course of dialogue this diversity must be respected, and the doctor should be wary of one-sided assessments and one-sided partisanship.

Techniques for the Family Interview

An active, structured interview is the precondition for the family dealing well with the problem situation. Different questioning techniques are useful to keep a balance between spontaneous statements of the family and a structured approach.

Direct Disease-Related Questions

Direct questions relate to facts, causes, and ways of behavior and experience that are easily accessible to the individual. Some examples include:

- "When did the first symptoms appear?"
- "How do relatives react to your illness?"
- "Who are you talking to about your symptoms? With whom preferably not?"
- "Who has the most fear of the disease?"

Indirect or Circular Questions

In the survey of family members about their own opinion of the disease, problem, or its impact, often interesting information is obtained if done in an indirect way. For example, the doctor asks, "Anna, what do you think of what your father thinks about the disease of your mother?"

Through circular questions, caregivers, but also family members, learn in a playful way about the different perspectives of each person. The questions invite the family member to enter into the minds of others and to define relationships consciously.

Hypothetical Questions

Hypothetical questions are also helpful. They allow the interviewer to introduce new options, try out new narratives, and therefore counteract the fear of change. Some examples of hypothetical questions include:

- "Suppose the migraine attacks of your wife would occur much less frequently, what would your wife and your family gain, what would this mean for the specific relationship in everyday life?"
- "Suppose one of your children would choose to return home to be there for the parents, who would be most likely to do that?"
- "Suppose we meet here again in 5 years, what do you think, are the parents still together? What will have changed? What will remain the same?"

Classification Questions

- "Who most likely shares the opinion of Paul regarding his mother's illness?"
- "Who the least?"

Percent Questions

- "What percentage do you think your complaints are the expression of physical illness, what percentage the expression of your current work and family problems?"

Solution-Oriented Questions

- "How often (how long, when) did the symptoms not occur?"
- "What did you and others do differently during those times?"

Pitfalls

- Confrontational statements usually lead to distrust and withdrawal of the family. Instead, the focus is on the emphasis and affirmation of the strengths and specifics of the family.
- Insufficient active structured interviewing: Unlike in individual contact with patients, couples or families reveal communication patterns that have formed in everyday life of the relationship. If the doctor does not structure the dialogue quickly and make it safe for each member to speak, there is a risk that old patterns are restaged, coalitions are formed, and individual family members may "check out" mentally from the conversation.

Cultural Aspects

While in Western cultures other family members are involved only in case of children and the elderly, the involvement of family is given in other cultures.

Asia

The Chinese culture is a kind of "high-context culture," where the people are highly dependent on each other and pay much attention to take care of each other. Familism embodies this culture and individuation is a rarely used exotic word in China. A family is identical to a small state and a state is identical to a large family. Therefore, all the interpersonal relations can be reduced to the following three orthodox basic rules from Confucianism:

- The monarch rules his minister.
- The father rules his sons.
- The man rules his wife.

Accordingly, the ruling and ruled people should follow five basic virtues:

- Humanity
- Responsibility
- Courtesy
- Wisdom
- Trustfulness

Confucianism requests a person to control himself and to obey social norm, to respect and to take care of other persons' interests at any time, to develop and maintain interpersonal relationship with a modest and polite attitude, and to improve himself through continuous practices. Familism is closely bound with moralism.

Outstanding Issues in Modern Chinese Families

Changes of family structure resulted in nuclear family becoming the main family pattern. Clan or large family has lost its social support functions. Women have equal legal and economic status in the family. But some families (especially husbands and their mothers) cannot adapt to such changes of two gender roles. Traditional values contradict the contemporary social reality, so that the so-called generation gap is very common within families. Anxiety about the uncertain future and fear of unsuccessful parenting makes the parent-children relationship much stickier and closer, which impacts the individuation process. A lot of children have to be reared and educated by grandparents or institutions as replacement parents. This is a very important factor for emotional and conduct disorders of adolescents, marriage crisis and sexual problems, neurosis and adaptation disorders. Stressful life styles and dysfunctional coping styles with stress are harmful for family life. Major hassles and burdens are making money, finding a job, purchasing apartments, rearing, and educating children. There is little time for family life and face-to-face communication.

What to Consider in the Family Dialogue?

In Asian families, the paternal authority is paramount. Thus, it is important in the beginning to treat the father with due respect and to ask him questions and to invite him to begin the dialogue or, with his permission, to involve the other family members in the conversation.

In more matriarchally oriented cultures, the grandmother should be treated with this kind of respect, even though she may seem rather withdrawn.

Examples of Culture-Related Family Problems

Cultural Differences Between Generations The parents are still stuck with traditional views and behaviors and have difficulties to adapt to the fast-paced changes in consumption and lifestyles in the context of globalization. The younger generation identifies quickly with new lifestyles and adopts new values, with a tendency to ignore old viewpoints, or even to despise them. Parents are confused and helpless, do not know how they should behave, and perceive a thread to their parental dominance and disciplinary power. This role confusion may be exacerbated when the children master the new media better and become the teachers of their parents.

The Roles of the Daughter-in-law in Asian Families In the traditional Hindu family, the focus is the mother-son relationship. The daughter-in-law has a subordinate position within the family. As a result, the daughter-in-law is often abused and punished, both physically and mentally, by the family members of the husband, especially, if she violates the rules of conduct with respect to the mother-in-law.

Violence Against Parents in Japan and China Often boys are brought up by their mother, while the father is absent due to his work or was perceived as weak and vulnerable. Violence against the mother or both parents is understood as an attempt to gain distance, mainly from the mother. As part of the one-child policy, this behavior is observed more and more frequently in China. As a small child, many boys are spoiled by their parents and grandparents and as a teenager they react with violence if their wants and needs are not met immediately.

Africa

In traditional African societies, extended families and associated social support that comes with it is a positive and protective factor against stressful life situations. The sense of belonging to the community and the presence of connections with other members of the community, ancestors, and the land, as well as collective responses to suffering, all somehow lift the burden of stress from an individual and distribute it to the various components of holistic living.

Latin America—The Low-Aged Patients

In cases of lower-age patients, doctor–patient relationship is mediated by the nearest relative. Nonetheless, a survey study carried out in the pediatric unit on effective participation of parents in the doctor–patient dialogue, demonstrated that there is a lack of satisfactory communicative relationship. The study evidenced that there is a need for training to improve doctors' communication skills as a tool for humanization and ethical action (Garrafa and Albuquerque 2001).

References

Carter B, McGoldrick M. The changing family life cycle: a framework for family therapy. Needham Heights: Allyn and Bacon; 1989.

Garrafa V, Albuquerque MC. Enfoque bioético de la comunicación en la relación médico-paciente em las unidades de terapia intensiva pediátricas. Acta Bioeth. 2001;7(2):355–367.

McDaniel S, Campbell TL, Hepworth J, Lorenz A. Family-oriented primary care. New York: Springer; 2005.

Chapter 8
Balint Group

Kurt Fritzsche, Frank Kuan-Yu Chen, Wei Jing, Gertrud Frahm and Sonia Diaz Monsalve

Case Study In the group, an internist reports that she had been annoyed lately about a patient suffering from diabetes mellitus, who treated her increasingly more arrogantly. Already when entering the office he welcomed her with condescension: "Well, how are you today, Doctor?" and "Today you don't look good." Now, she gets annoyed by just seeing the patient.

(Continued)

K. Fritzsche (✉) · S. D. Monsalve
Department of Psychosomatic Medicine and Psychotherapy, University Medical Center, Hauptstr. 8, 79104 Freiburg, Germany
e-mail: kurt.fritzsche@uniklinik-freiburg.de

S. D. Monsalve
e-mail: sonia.diaz-monsalve@uniklinik-freiburg.de

F. K.-Y. Chen
Division of Psychosomatic Medicine, Taipei City Psychiatric Center, Taipei City Hospital, No. 309 Song-De Road, Taipei 11080, Taiwan
e-mail: kychen@ms4.hinet.net

W. Jing
Department of Psychological Medicine, Peking Union Medical College Hospital, 1 Shuaifuyuan, Dongcheng District, Beijing 100730, China
e-mail: weijing@pumch.cn

G. Frahm
Department of Human Sciences, Federal University of Paraná, R. Gal. Carneiro, 460, Curitiba, PR 80060-150, Brazil
e-mail: gfrahm@uol.com.br

K. Fritzsche et al. (eds.), *Psychosomatic Medicine,* DOI 10.1007/978-1-4614-1022-5_8,

Definition

Balint groups are case studies with particular emphasis on the doctor–patient relationship. A doctor presents a patient who is on his/her mind for various reasons. The group reflects on the doctor–patient relationship from various angles, which allows the doctor to obtain the views of others and perceive interfering unconscious influences as well as his/her own contributions to the problem. This creates a new understanding and a new level of relationship. These new perspectives lead doctors to a better understanding of themselves and the patient and provide the impetus for a more satisfactory course of treatment.

What is a Balint Group?

- Its primary task is to promote further understanding and thought about the relationship between clinicians and patients.
- The method is an exploration of the relationship between a particular clinician and a particular patient.
- A Balint group is the opportunity to explore in depth a clinical case that presents a puzzle.
- It allows for professionals from different backgrounds to get to know and understand each other and their work.

Relevance

A good doctor–patient relationship is the dominant factor for a successful and satisfactory treatment. For diagnosis and treatment, it is important on the one hand to observe the behavior of the patient exactly; on the other hand, the doctor can also get important insights by exploring his/her own thoughts, feelings, and behavior impulses.

Doctors are important attachment figures for the patient, to whom positive and negative thoughts, feelings, hopes, and desires are transferred. The doctor must be aware of this, without interpreting the thoughts and feelings. The patient's behavior and feelings influence the doctor's thoughts, feelings, and actions and may, in extreme cases, confuse him/her and make him/her unable to act. The doctor, too, has his/her emotional developmental history with strengths and weaknesses, which he/she must recognize.

Patients who feel understood holistically in terms of a biopsychosocial anamnesis are happier and show better compliance. Importantly, their treatment will therefore cost less money.

Theory

Historical Background

Michael Balint was born on 3 December 1896 in Budapest as the son of a general practitioner (GP). After studying medicine, he trained as a psychoanalyst. Very early on, he became interested in psychosomatic diseases and focused on the importance of adequate psychological understanding in the medical profession. He wanted to raise awareness in GPs that mental processes play a role in disease symptoms in addition to organic causes. The focus was on the close observation of the doctor–patient relationship and the desired effects and side effects thereof. In his collaboration with GPs, he wanted to empower them to consciously create relationships with their patients and to use these as a healing force. His best-known book is *The Doctor, His Patient and the Illness,* published in 1957 (Balint 2000).

Objectives of Participation

Case Example The doctor introduces a young female patient with severe anorexia nervosa, who drives him to despair and devaluates any treatment suggestion. Following this, the group having addressed the patient for some time, discussed various aspects of her behavior, and also made proposals for treatment, the presenting physician was included again: All that was said was of no use to him. It would not help him at all. He did not feel understood at all.

These were exactly the words with which he introduced the patient initially. Now, he can sense how the patient feels with her illness and the various treatment attempts. He felt her weakness, her insecurity, and her desperation. From the perspective of the patient, he was able to express his wishes to the group and to accept the education proposals of the group better.

There is a parallel process between the presented doctor–patient relationship and the relationship between the presenting doctor and the Balint group. If it is possible, therefore, for the doctor to empathize with the patient as a person with all the accompanying feelings, then he/she will succeed from this perspective to understand the patient and the interaction between him and the patient better. The concept of Balint group is specifically targeted at raising awareness of this countertransference phenomenon, the patient initiates at the doctor. Feelings of countertransference can be used professionally as valuable information on diagnostic perception and understanding of the patient. This may develop into further therapeutic interventions.

Countertransference

In psychoanalysis, *countertransference* is a form of transference in which the therapist responds to the patient and, in turn, directs his/her own feelings, prejudices, expectations, and desires onto the patient. The therapist leaves his/her neutral position for different motives—usually temporarily. For this reason, in the early days of psychoanalysis countertransference was considered a disruptive influence the therapist must become aware of and resolve. Modern psychoanalysis sees the feelings of the therapist toward the patient as a "sounding board," by which he/she gains information about the patient.

Objectives of the Balint Group

- Openness for both interview content and one's own reactions, in the form of feelings, fantasies, and bodily sensations evoked by the interview
- Practice in better listening and patience
- More sensitivity for the presence of an emotional disorder or psychosomatic problem
- Anxiety-free dealing with the patient's emotional and social problems
- Better understanding of the interactions between doctor and patient
- Application of this understanding in diagnostics and therapy
- Altered attitude and altered behavior of the doctor toward the patient treated
- Better understanding of unconscious processes
- Emotional relief and prevention of burnout
- Recognition of doctor's own feelings toward problem patients (counter transference)
- The doctor develops a more analytic way of thinking
- The doctor is more aware of his/her personal influence on the patient

Environment and the Course of a Balint Group

A Balint group is made up of 8–12 participants. The group leader is a psychoanalytic psychotherapist, familiar with group processes and has experience in the management of Balint groups. The group meets on a regular basis. A session lasts approximately one and a half hours.

The presenting doctor describes a doctor–patient relationship from memory, without using notes or file cards. An experience and emotional impression arises of the speaker, the patient, and their relationship with one another. The participants hearing this report then give their impression, their feelings, and their fantasies about what they have heard. This results in a complex image of the doctor–patient relationship

Table 8.1 Questions of the group leader for the participants of a Balint group

What do you think the patient was feeling at that moment?
What kind of person is the patient?
What do you know about his/her life situation, his present family, and his family of origin?
What feelings does this patient elicit in us?
How does the patient shape his doctor to his needs and possibilities and vice versa?
Where is there an underlying "disrupted fit" between the patient and his environment and how is this reflected?
How do you think the patient sees his doctor and what does he think of him?
Why did the doctor behave as he did in this situation and what did he want to achieve with this behavior?
Is there something the patient is missing in the doctor and perhaps in his life as well?
What feelings does this patient elicit in us?
How do you think the patient sees his doctor and what does he think of him?
Why did the doctor behave as he did in this situation and what did he want to achieve with this behavior?
Is there something the patient is missing in the doctor and perhaps in his life as well?

that the speaker can observe quietly from a distance, without speaking. He/she obtains suggestions for a new point of view; blind spots are illuminated. The clinician recognizes his/her effect on the patient and his/her own behavioral pattern. Balint work enables on the one hand some self-experience for the doctor and, on the other hand, the doctor learns to keep not only the disease but the patient's entire personality in view. Treatment proceeds in a more relaxed atmosphere. The patient and the doctor are more comfortable.

Tasks of the Group Leader

The group leader's task is to make these basic premises part of the doctor–patient relationship presented. In Table 8.1, there are some questions that may be asked.

Practice

Case Study Follow-up The group will discuss how the annoyance of the fellow doctor about the patient is to be understood. One idea was to understand the patient's behavior as an unconscious attempt not to have to respond to unpleasant topics. Encouraged by the free discussion in the group the internist shared her fantasies about the patient: She experienced him like an overflowing trash can on a narrow staircase an elderly gentleman had to struggle with. This was, however, quite contrary to the lively and cheerful entering of the patient into the treatment room.

At the next visit, the internist was brave enough to show the patient the contradiction: "Amazingly, Mr. Miller, you come in here quite cheerful but at the same time I have in my head the picture of an elderly man struggling with a trash can." The patient then got a very wry face and said, "Have we ever talked about my wife, how she constantly tantalizes me with her cleanliness compulsion, and how she is trying to make me part of her cleaning mania?" He also said that he often eats sweets out of frustration, and he was now embarrassed to talk about it.

At the next meeting with the patient, from the beginning, there was a good atmosphere between doctor and patient. The blood sugar levels have improved over the course of the following week.

Sculpture Work and Balint Group

Sculpture work is a method in couple and family therapy. A sculpture of a system (family, hospital team) enables access to tensions, conflicts, and previously unseen positive and negative relationships within the system. After presenting a case, the presenting colleague first selects persons from among the group participants as representatives of those involved in the case and positions them in the room. He/she plays the role of the doctor. The symptoms or the disease are also personified by a participant. This makes the closeness or distance in the relationship clear.

The trainer supports this process by asking the positioned participants, "Whom do you see? How do you feel standing there?" The trainer can intensify the process by further questions about physical and emotional perceptions, by requesting the person to make a typical gesture, or to say a sentence spontaneously. After the presenter has arranged the representatives of his/her case, he/she is only an observer and lets the trainer and the representatives do and say what they wish. The amazing thing about this method is that, from where they stand, the positioned representatives have access to the feelings and relationships of the families—or team members—involved. The goal is to recognize and dissolve snags between the family members or in the team and to find a new order in which every person is comfortable in their position.

The creation of a sculpture by the Balint group may be included as another way to help the group to visualize and facilitate a new perspective on the doctor's relationship with the patient, and the environment of both the doctor and the patient. This work clearly shows that the encounter of the doctor and the patient is not a two-character play, and the impact of the family, the staff, and the environment plays a crucial role in dealing with each other and thus in the diagnosis and the treatment or therapy. This environment may include the family and significant relationships of the patient, the patient's and the doctor's lifestyle and financial circumstances and the clinical situation in which the consultation takes place. From our experience, this is a common feature in Balint groups around the world. This impact can be more clearly demonstrated by the group when they create a group sculpture. The emotional experience of sculpture work is used for a better understanding of the dynamics of relationship formation (Otten 2007, 2012).

Cultural Aspects

Asia

The introduction of sculpture work as a modifying element of the Balint group enabled a symbolic test activity for the participants (see also Chap. 17). Using sculpture work led to dissolution of the rigid structures and a solution which was comfortable for all representatives. Introduction of the sculpture in the Balint group work arose from previous experience in Vietnam and Laos: In these two countries, more than in China, it is not customary to speak directly about personal feelings. This was repeatedly confirmed in the first discussions of Balint group work with their future trainers. The participants would feel overtaxed or intruded upon by the instruction to freely express their thoughts, fantasies, and feelings. Our experience with the classical Balint work appeared initially to confirm this. The situation appeared completely different when sculpting was introduced. The participants became completely absorbed in their roles, spoke of their fears, their anger, and their sadness, and identified with the person they represented. In this way, the sculpture gained in vivacity and dynamics. Hidden conflicts became emotionally palpable; hints for possible solutions were perceptible. The doctor-as-person was always represented, was part of the system, and contributed by a change of position to a decrease in the symptoms of the patients.

Latin America

Within the most different resources and techniques available for health professional development used in the Latin American continent, Balint groups are becoming more and more part of doctors' training programs. This is noticeable due to the increase of research interest, from the amount of advertisement for Balint group training short courses offered within and outside the university realms, as well as other bibliography productions (Missenard et al. 1994).

Balint group is also used for the health professional development. Balint group work might be considered a beginning for the establishment of the "espaço para a palavra" (space for the word), even in cases where working conditions are not in favor of this possibility (Brandt 2009). The "espaço de palavra" (space of the word) creates an adequate group atmosphere and the possibility of the doctor to acquire a differentiated professional status with more respect, more adequate autonomous creativity, and more assertive decision-making capability. The professionals submitted to Balint group work showed more autonomy in the relationship with leaders within and outside the working context, with an added quality of a humanistic approach whenever occupying leadership positions. Moreover, Balint group work has shown to be efficient, whenever used in neutral environment without the influence of the working organization, for the development of empathy; thus, promoting prevalence of humanistic ethics. Brand's findings evidenced that it is possible to reeducate leaders so as to turn them into democratic humanists to become healthy models of identification as outcome of Balint group work.

References

Balint M. The doctor, his patient and the illness, 2nd edition. London: Pitman: 1964. 3rd Millenium edition: Edinburgh: Churchill Livingstone; 2000.

Brandt JA. Grupo Balint: o recomeço para os líderes. Tese de Doutorado ao Instituto de Psicologia da Universidade de São Paulo. São Paulo. http://www.teses.usp.br/teses/disponiveis/47/47134/tde-22042010-151832/pt-br.php. 2009.

Missenard A, Balint M, Gelly R, Gosling R, Turquet PM, Sapir M. A experiê ncia Balint: historia e atualidade. São Paulo: Casa do psicólogo. 1994. ISBN: 85-84141-02-8.

Otten, H. Balintarbeit mit Skulptur. [Balint work with sculpture]. In: Häfner S, editor. Die Balintgruppe, [The Balint group]. Köln: Deutscher Ärzteverlag; 2007. pp. 89–94.

Otten, H. Professionelle Beziehungen—Theorie und Praxis der Balintgruppenarbeit. [Professional relationships—theories and practice of Balint groups]. Heidelberg: Springer; 2012.

Part III
Recognition and Treatment of Most Common Clinical Presentations

Chapter 9
Depressive Disorders

Kurt Fritzsche, Wei Jing, Frank Kuan-Yu Chen, Kim Viet Nguyen, Van Tuan Nguyen, Catherine Abbo, Gertrud Frahm and Sonia Diaz Monsalve

Case Study Mr. Miller, a 30-year-old Law student, visits his general practitioner (GP) because of tinnitus. He complains about chronic fatigue and vertigo for some time. He is having a hard time coping with his difficulties to

K. Fritzsche (✉) · S. D. Monsalve
Department of Psychosomatic Medicine and Psychotherapy, University Medical Center, Hauptstr. 8, 79104 Freiburg, Germany
e-mail: kurt.fritzsche@uniklinik-freiburg.de

S. D. Monsalve
e-mail: sonia.diaz-monsalve@uniklinik-freiburg.de

W. Jing
Department of Psychological Medicine, Peking Union Medical College Hospital, 1 Shuaifuyuan, Dongcheng District, 100730 Beijing, China
e-mail: weijing@pumch.cn

F. K.-Y. Chen
Division of Psychosomatic Medicine, Taipei City Psychiatric Center, Taipei City Hospital, No. 309 Song-De Road, 11080 Taipei, Taiwan
e-mail: kychen@ms4.hinet.net

K. V. Nguyen · V. T. Nguyen
Department of Psychiatry, Hanoi Medical University, No. 1, Ton That Tung Street, Dong Da District, Hanoi, Vietnam
e-mail: drnkimviet@yahoo.com

National Institute of Mental Health, Bach Mai Hospital, No. 78, Giai Phong Road, Dong Da District, Hanoi, Vietnam

V. T. Nguyen
e-mail: nvtuannimhvn@hmu.edu.vn

C. Abbo
Department of Psychiatry, Makerere University College of Health Sciences and Mulago National Referral and Teaching Hospital, Mulago Hill Road, 7072 Kampala, Uganda
e-mail: cathyabbo@chs.mak.ac.ug, cathya180@gmail.com

G. Frahm
Department of Human Sciences, Federal University of Paraná, R. Gal. Carneiro, 460, Curitiba, PR 80060-150, Brazil
e-mail: gfrahm@uol.com.br

K. Fritzsche et al. (eds.), *Psychosomatic Medicine*, DOI 10.1007/978-1-4614-1022-5_9,

Table 9.1 Depressive symptoms at four levels

Behavior	Feelings	Body	Thoughts
Powerless and bent posture, slowed movements, sad facial expression, sometimes like a mask and stony faced, soft, slow, and monotonous speech, reduced activity with limited radius of movement	Dependent, sad, hopeless, helpless, alone and anxious, hostile mood toward others, inner restlessness, feelings of isolation, feelings of guilt	Physical weakness, apathy, loss of appetite, sleeping problems, reactions to weather changes, increased sensitivity to pain, loss of libido, multiple vegetative complaints such as pressure in the head, gastric complaints and impaired digestion	Determined by a negative attitude toward himself and the future, pessimism, permanent self-criticism, lack of self-confidence, concentration problems, impaired memory, anticipation of catastrophes, ideas of hopelessness and purposelessness of his own life, suicidal thoughts, expectation of punishment, delusions such as impending poverty, and compulsive high level of demand on himself

concentrate because he is preparing for his state examination. He can only focus for a short time, and then his thoughts get off–track; he is not being able to really think anything through because every thought starts straying again. Mr. Miller then gets up because he cannot sit still; he feels too restless. He hardly goes out anymore, is not cultivating his friendships lately, is afraid to face up to the questions of whether he is making progress with his studies, and blaming himself enough already anyway; everything seems to be hopeless to him.

Mr. Miller grew up in a very strict and achievement-oriented home. When he was 13 years old, his father lost his job, a shock that his father has never overcome. He started drinking and withdrew more and more. One year later, Mr. Miller found his father on the roof beam where he committed suicide. Mr. Miller does not talk about this incident, although he sometimes still sees the pictures in his dreams. In secret, he is reproaching his mother for not being there enough for his father; for him, his father might still be alive if there had been more empathy.

(Continued)

Definition

As apparent from the case study, depressive symptoms are expressed at various levels (Table 9.1).

Relevance

Depression is the most frequent mental disorder. Over time, every sixth person suffers from depression, and the risk is twice as high for women than for men. Depression can negatively affect the treatment of physical illnesses or can even be the cause for somatization. Despite their high relevance, depressions are scarcely identified by GPs or consulting physicians. Nearly half of all depressive disorders remain undetected. This is particularly dramatic because of the high suicide risk.

Theory

Symptoms

Main Symptoms

- Dejected, depressive mood
- Lack of interest and/or joylessness, even in otherwise pleasant events
- Apathy, easily exhausted

Secondary Symptoms

- Reduced concentration and attention span
- Reduced self-esteem and self-confidence
- Feelings of guilt and worthlessness
- Negative and pessimistic future perspectives
- Suicidal thoughts/acts
- Sleep disruptions
- Reduced/increased appetite

The inclusion criteria for a depressive episode are met when several of the above-mentioned symptoms are present for at least 2 weeks.

Diagnostic Categories

The most frequent affective disorders are depressive episodes (ICD-10: F32, F33) and dysthymia (ICD-10: F34.1). Manic episodes (ICD-10: F30) and bipolar affective disorders (ICD-10: F31) are described in textbooks on psychiatry.

Table 9.2 Checklist depressive episode (ICD-10 F)

Guiding symptoms	
Gloom, abjectness	□
Loss of interest and/or pleasure	□
Decrease of motivation/strong signs of fatigue	□
Additional symptoms	
Impaired concentration and attention	□
Impaired self-esteem and self-confidence	□
Feelings of guilt/worthlessness	□
Negative and pessimistic future perspectives	□
Suicidal thoughts and actions	□
Sleeping problems (early wakening)	□
Decreased appetite—weight—libido	□
Psychotic symptoms	
Delusions (catastrophes, sins, impoverishness)	□
Hallucinations (accusing/defaming voices)	□
Psychomotor impairment—stupor	□

To be treated depressive episode: minimum of two main symptoms and two additional symptoms, ≥ 2 weeks

Depressive Episodes (ICD-10: F32; see Table 9.2)

A differentiation is made between mild, moderate, and serious depressive episodes:

- *Mild*: Two main symptoms and two secondary symptoms (F32.0).
- *Moderate*: Two main symptoms and 3–4 secondary symptoms (F32.1).
- *Serious*: Three main symptoms and ≥ 4 secondary symptoms (F32.2).

The presence of other emotional disorders (i.e., addiction, anxiety disorders, and eating disorders) is a risk factor for chronic depressions and suicidal tendencies.

Dysthymia (ICD-10: F 34.1)

This disorder was formerly called neurotic depression. The characteristics are:

- Long-lasting depressive mood which is not expressed in a way that the criteria for a depressive episode are met (Fig. 9.1).
- Onset in early adulthood. Duration of several years, sometimes lifelong.

Typical symptoms: fatigue, sleeping problems, easily exhausted, brooding, complaining, and feeling of inadequacy.

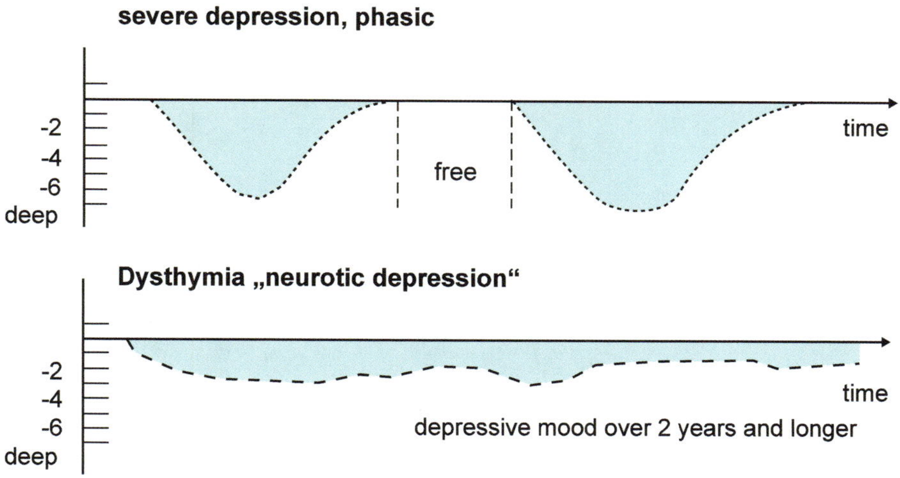

Fig. 9.1 Comparison between "severe depression" and "dysthymia"

Differential Diagnosis

Adjustment Disorders

Depressive symptoms also are found as a reaction to severe psychosocial stress or certain life events, e.g., diagnosis of a life-threatening illness. A difference is made between short *depressive reactions*, which do not last longer than 1 month, and longer depressive reactions, which do not last longer than 2 years (ICD-10: F 43).

Depression/Grief

The illness depression must be differentiated from *sadness* or *grief*. Sadness or grief is a normal feeling like rage, joy, or fear and belongs to the basic human emotions. The capacity for sadness is biologically designed. Feelings of sadness are usually transient. Sadness or grief is often the result of the loss of a significant other. The feelings of dependency, self-doubt, hopelessness, and helplessness also occur in a depression, but not with the same intensity, and the loss of self-esteem is usually not as drastic. In contrary to a depression, sadness can often be interrupted by positive, pleasant activities and events. Grief is transient with confident future perspectives and the maintained capacity to seek help and support. Grieving takes time. The development of depression or physical complaints without organic findings (somatization) are promoted by unsuccessful and stifled grieving.

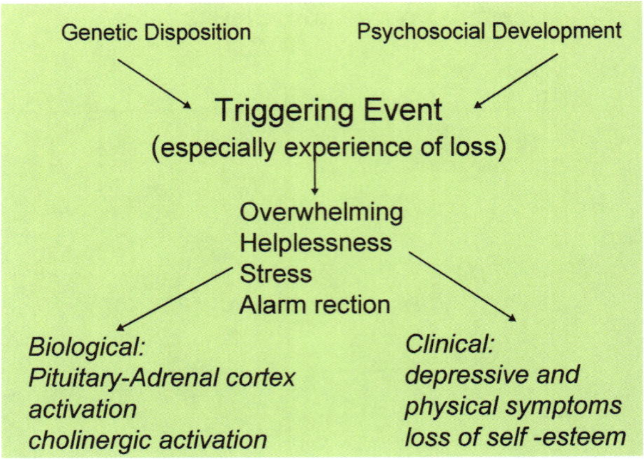

Fig. 9.2 The biopsychosocial model of depression

Frequency and Course

According to a European study (Wittchen et al. 2011), affective disorders have a 12-month prevalence of 7.8 %. Here, major depression is the most common diagnosis—6.9 % of the EU population per year is diagnosed with this disorder. 0.9 % is attributable to a diagnosis of bipolar disorder. In a previous study, it was found that approximately half of all patients with depression for the first time suffered a further depressive episode during subsequent years. The probability for another illness after the second time was 70 %, and that after the third episode was 90 %. The difference in course between a recurrent depressive disorder and dysthymia is shown above.

Biopsychosocial Model of the Onset of Depressions

According to the biopsychosocial model, several factors are involved in the onset and manifestation of depressions (Fig. 9.2), whereby their severity differs depending on the individual.

Genetic Disposition

Depressions often occur in families. If both parents suffered from depressions, the risk of the illness is approximately 50 % in the children.

Neurochemical and Neuroendocrinological Correlating Distress Reaction

The *serotonin theory* assumes that a low serotonin level strongly affects the neural activities of other neurochemical systems and leads to mania or depression. The antidepressive effect of antidepressant drugs are attributed to an increase in the availability of serotonin and noradrenalin in the synaptic cleft.

Depression is a potent stressor. It leads to an activation of the hypothalamus-pituitary-adrenal cortex axis with a subsequent excessive *cortisol production*.

Cognitions

Cognitions are all mental processes associated with perception, imagination, memory, learning, thinking, and judgment. Cognitions may elicit feelings and moods. Depressive patients have a pessimistic view of themselves, the world, and the future (*negative triad*). Because of negative life experiences, they have acquired negative convictions and action patterns (schemata), which lead to cognitive distortions in stressful situations, for example, arbitrary conclusions and selective perception.

The *concept of learned helplessness* is cited as an example. In their biographies, there are repeated uncontrollable traumatic events that these patients had to passively accept, with no possibility of developing avoidance and coping reactions. The learned helplessness leads to the expectation that subsequent negative experiences cannot be controlled either. One effect is that the actual given possibilities of influence are not used and that the response is depressive withdrawal. In addition, the patient always looks to himself for the reason for failure.

Psychosocial Stress

Before the first occurrence of a depression, there are usually typical stress situations: interpersonal conflicts, loss of prestige or insults, threatened or finally accomplished separations, or death of a significant other.

A common characteristic of these events is the *threat* or the *loss of interpersonal bonds*. People who experienced separation more often or a serious endangerment of their predominant protective relationships in the first years of life show a long-lasting sensitization of their biological stress response to conflicts, separations, or losses in adulthood. These people also show an elevated risk for depression. Critical psychosocial stress leads to a greater and longer lasting alarming of their stress system.

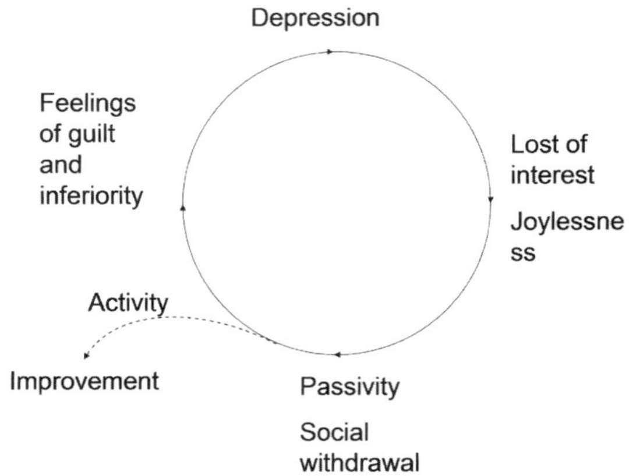

Fig. 9.3 Vicious circle model of depression

Psychodynamics

Because of the fear of more separations and losses, these people have developed a *high degree of responsibility and sense of duty*, and they expect great things from themselves to satisfy others. So they hope to be needed by others and to offset their love deficit. At the same time, this behavior serves to maintain their self-esteem. Their own needs, annoyance, rage, and disappointment are initially repulsed and then directed at themselves in self-blame, self-accusation, and attempted suicide.

Communicative Function—the Vicious Circle Model

The depressive patient is caught in a vicious circle during the depressive episodes (Fig. 9.3). The loss of interest and joylessness as a result of the depression leads to withdrawal and passivity. Friends are neglected; favored hobbies are not appealing anymore. Usually, it is still possible to fulfill duties such as going to work or taking care of the children, but all these tasks are performed carelessly and with little engagement. This passivity amplifies the existing feelings of guilt and inferiority; the depressive person observes his own behavior but cannot change it. He is condemning himself for what he is doing or rather not doing. The crestfallen mood and hopelessness are thereby increased. The patient resignedly reacts on impulses and suggestions from his environment, friends, and supporters in an inner dialog: “You are right, but I’m not worth it that you are spending your time with me, it is hopeless, and I’m not able to do anything reasonable anyway.”

Practice

Recognition

Most depressive patients can be identified with two questions. However, there are some patients in which depression is hidden behind physical symptoms.

Practical Tip "Diagnostic Questions for Depression" (Arroll et al. 2003)
"Have you often felt crestfallen, sad, gloomy, or hopeless within the last month?"

"Have you lost interest and pleasure in things that you normally love to do within the last month?"

Table 9.2 sets out the central symptom areas that need to be scanned to detect depression.

Case Study (Continued) "Recognition"
T: "Mr. Miller, you have described a couple of problems to me: chronic fatigue, difficulties to concentrate, and vertigo. I will refer you to an ENT specialist for the tinnitus. These symptoms often are connected to stress though, are you undergoing something like that?"
P: "Yes, I'm about to take my exams; at least I'm trying, but I guess I won't make it."
T: "Exams."
P: "Yes, the state examination, but this is rather difficult; actually, I don't need to take it."
T: "Hmm, you have a lot of stress due to the exam and can't even imagine anymore that this could work out."
P: (Looking down) "Exactly."
T: "What is it like in other areas: friends, hobbies?" (*Diagnostic clarification*)
P: "I'm not doing anything at the moment. If I can, I'm studying, and otherwise, I'm too tired, or I don't feel like it."
T: "When you think of last month, have you felt crestfallen, sad, gloomy, or hopeless?" (*Screening question* 1)
T: "Yes, sure. Mainly gloomy and hopeless. I'm just really in over my head right now."
T: "And what about your interest and pleasure in things that you like to do last month?" (*Screening question* 2)
P: "I liked to go out with friends in the past, but I think they don't want to go out with me anymore; I'm just a turnoff."

(Continued)

Basic Therapeutic Attitude

Depressive people are so weakened and wounded in their self-respect and self-esteem that they react to any kind of disruption in interpersonal relationships. The physician's key task is primarily to listen patiently to the patient and accept his complaints *without* giving him *premature encouragement*. The physician must dare to accompany the patient even if this shortly leads to the experience of the depressive person's entire misery. The paralyzing feeling might be even amplified, and the impulse to do something grows stronger. The central problem of the conversation is to keep the balance between accompanying, activating, and informing and not to get involved into a tug-of-war in which the physician is trying to help while the patient is using his depression as a defense.

Basic Intervention

Accompanying—Activating—Informing

How can you approach depressive patients when all well-meaning advice is lost in the whirlpool of hopelessness? Basically, the patient is *accompanied* at first. The hopelessness is not euphemized but is reflected. So the patient is experiencing something rare: he is being taken seriously in what he says, and nobody is immediately speaking to the contrary. At the same time, the doctor signals the patient that it is possible to talk about the feelings of heaviness and to bear them up—an experience that is not leaving the depressive person utterly alone anymore. Accompanying a patient usually has an interesting effect rather soon: the depressive person cannot argue against the physician anymore and cannot convince him of the impossibility of his suggestion, and the patient is basically thrown on his own resources.

From this feeling, the question usually arises as to what should happen next. The physician can seize upon these small signals. It shows a minimum of *activity* that the patient is asking a future-related question. This activity needs to be supported and to be emphasized. Another activating conversational method is to strengthen the nondepressive part of the patient's personality. Whenever the patient is talking about his former self, this can be emphasized as the actual personality, but it should always be hereby accepted that this personality is not available at the moment. The generalization that the depressive person is bad is overcome by these interventions, and the episode character of the disorder is underlined.

If the patient is willing to take on a little responsibility, the physician can start *to give information* and support. It is important to clarify that the symptoms are part of the depressive disorders and that depression can be treated successfully. As depressive patients are usually able to fulfill given tasks, structuring is helpful. The physician needs to keep in mind that the structure does not include an overstrain, relaxation phases are strictly limited in time, and relaxation is not gained by sleeping but, if possible, by exercise. In discussing the daily routine, the positive activities can be emphasized again.

Case Study (Continued) T: "Ok, your friends don't feel like going out with you anymore." (*Accompanying*)
P: (crestfallen) "Yes, I wouldn't feel like going out with me either. I'm just spoiling the mood anyway."
T: "Actually nobody can stand you like that." (*Accompanying*)
P: "Exactly." (Pause) "Actually, I've been a pretty entertaining guy, but this is all gone."
T: "I understand, you are actually a social person, but you don't recognize this side of yourself anymore right now." (*Seizing on the nondepressive personality*)
P: "Yes, gone, like blown out."
T: "This side simply disappeared, is gone." (*Accompanying*)
P: (Pause) "Do you think I can get it back?" (*Shows activity*)
T: "When you think about it, the question arises: can I become my old self again?" (*Activating*)
P: "My old self, I don't think so but maybe a little. You think that works?"
T: "Yes, I do. What you are suffering from is a depression; that is an illness which can be treated." (Informing)

Practical Tip "Green Recipe"

1. Examples of the diverse possibilities that depression can manifest itself include lack of motivation, lack of energy, rapid exhaustion, lack of interest and anhedonia, guilt, anxiety, feelings of incompetence, lack of appetite, weight loss, sleep disturbances, somatic complaints, and social withdrawal.
2. If you suffer from depression, then you are not the only one: About 10 % of the population will at some point in the life go through a major depression.
3. Even if you lost hope: Depression can be treated successfully with consistent treatment; the chances of healing by drug treatment or by cognitive behavior therapy are good.
4. Avoid prolonged retreat with excessive rumination (plan distracting activities) and avoid morning sleep. Try to maintain a regular daily routine.
5. Make sure that you comply with general rules for reducing stress: Stick exactly to sufficient time for relaxation and change, break planning, leisure activities, not too many stressing activities at the same time (e.g., moving, changing jobs, etc.), and healthy nutrition (→ doctor).
6. Check whether there were significant changes in your life before you became depressed (professional or private), losses, failure experiences, interpersonal conflicts, excessive demands, relocation, or change of job and discuss these with your doctor.

Psychopharmaceutical Treatment

With *mild* and *moderate* depressive disorders, psychopharmaceutical treatment may be used as a supplement to psychotherapeutic treatment. However, it has been found that a psychotherapeutic treatment of the initial manifestation reduces the risk of a second depression later, whereas sheer drug treatment of the first depression shows a tendency of an increased risk to suffer from another depression later.

In serious cases, treatment with antidepressive psychopharmaceuticals in combination with psychotherapy is absolutely indicated. It must be noted that the patient also has to be informed that there is a latency of at least 2 weeks for all antidepressants to show an effect, whereas side effects may occur immediately. Medication should be continued for approximately 6–9 months. In case of recurrent depressions, a long-term prophylaxis is indicated.

The *antidepressants* can be attributed to three groups according to clinical-practical aspects, depending on the active ingredients, and to certain main indications.

- *Energy-increasing* antidepressants such as the selective serotonin-reuptake inhibitors (SSRI)
- *Sedating* antidepressants: Mirtazepin, a specific serotonergic antidepressant.
- *Others* are Venlaflaxine, Duloxetine

The prescription of psychopharmaceuticals requires a trusting doctor–patient relationship, which serves also to support medication compliance. Particularly in difficult phases of the treatment, for example, right at the beginning when the desired antidepressive effect is not yet apparent, but side effects occur to impair well-being, it is crucial that the patient feels taken seriously, when he, for instance, complains about side effects. The physician also should not take it lightly if the complaints do not match the typical spectrum of side effects.

The efficacy of antidepressive *drug therapy* is particularly well-documented in the acute phase. Psychotherapy is superior to drug treatment in the long term. Antidepressants help in 70–80 % of the cases. The average effect latency of 14 days must be considered. Antidepressants have an impact on the central transmitter substances, especially serotonin, noradrenalin, and dopamine.

What to Do in Case of Suicidality?

Recognition

Suicidality often exists—especially with elderly depressive patients—for months and is considered a taboo for the outside ("you don't talk about such things") and for the inside, that is, the patient mostly does not entertain these wishes but is overwhelmed by these pressing thoughts at other times which are experienced partly as alien to the patient's personality. Frequently, the patient seeks medical attendance after such a suicidal crisis (Table 9.3).

Table 9.3 Risk factors of suicidal actions

Patients with chronic progressive painful conditions
Isolation, confinement, breaking off contacts
Recent loss
Suicidal actions in the past
Suicide in the family (biological factors and learning-history factors, identification)
Certain emotional disorders (bipolar disorder, melancholic and psychotic depression, schizophrenia)

Table 9.4 Question catalogue in case of suicidality

Have you recently thought about killing yourself?
Often?
Have you had to think about it without wanting to?
Have suicidal thoughts forced themselves on you?
Could you ward these thoughts off?
Do you have concrete ideas or plans about how you would do it?
Have you made any arrangements?
Is there something that makes your life worth living?
Have you talked to anyone about your intention to commit suicide?
Have you ever attempted suicide?
Has anyone in your family or a friend or acquaintance committed suicide?

If a depressive disorder is assumed, the still unmentioned symptoms of a depression shall be specifically questioned. Death wishes or suicidal thoughts have to be implicitly questioned. The patient mostly does not entertain these wishes but is overwhelmed by these pressing thoughts at other times which are experienced partly as alien to the patient's personality (Table 9.4).

Practical Tip "Recognition"

Typical patient comments are:

- I may as well pack it all in.
- There is no point in that anymore anyway!
- I do not know anyway what else to do at home ... there is only one thing left to do.
- It would have been better to die of this heart attack.

The patient can usually only talk about these shameful thoughts that are a taboo if the physician is indicating that this is a common and human subject and that he has no issues with it at all. It is important to identify suicidality to estimate the suicidal endangerment and to openly and concretely seize upon suicidality.

A limitation of emotions, interpersonal relationships, and his scope occurs with a depressive, suicidal person. This limitation is usually noticeable from the outside. Close friends or family members realize a change in behavior; the person concerned is more and more withdrawn or makes certain insinuations.

Table 9.5 The stepped-care-model

The stepped-care-model
Step 1: All known and suspected presentations of depression
Assessment, support, psychoeducation, active monitoring, and referral for further assessment and interventions
Step 2: Mild to moderate depression
Psychosocial interventions, medication, and referral for further assessment and interventions
Step 3: Severe and complex depression
Combined treatments of high-intensity psychological interventions and medication
Crisis service
Inpatient care

Every insinuation has to be taken very seriously. The feeling of endangerment of a patient, which the physician experiences during the conversation, has a special character and importance. The opportunity for an open conversation about this difficult and highly ambivalent subject, which is extremely charged with feelings of guilt and shame, is a relief for the patient if this conversation is conducted in an understanding and emphatic way and not like an interrogation. The following question catalogue (Table 9.5) can serve as an orientation for such an open and impartial conversation.

The No-Suicide Contract

The medical-therapeutic interview should be completed preferably with a no-suicide contract. A prerequisite for this is that the patient is capable of making arrangements. The doctor can assess this based on the previous conversation:

- How readily does the patient talk about his suicidal intentions and the underlying problems of life?
- Is the doctor able to make an emotional contact with the patient?
- Has the patient the cognitive ability to reflect on his/her situation?

Practical Tip Example of wording
A: I would like to ask you, first orally and then in writing, to guarantee that you would not hurt yourself.

I would like you to say the following sentence aloud and to look at myself:

I guarantee that I am not going to kill myself either deliberately or through negligence, no matter what happens and how I feel. If I have thoughts of death, I will check into the emergency room of the psychiatric clinic. I undertake to comply with this until tomorrow morning at 8 o' clock.

After the patient has said these words, the doctor reaffirms the contract with a handshake and clear eye contact. If the patient is reluctant to say these words, speaks indistinctly, is not emotionally involved, and avoids eye contact, the doctor asks the patient to repeat the sentence with a loud voice and participation from the heart and to look him in the eye. If the patient is unable to comply despite verbally assuring otherwise, there is a significant suicide risk and an indication for hospitalization.

As an additional assurance, the doctor can have a written contract, having the patient sign it and hand him/her a copy. The wording of the contract depends on the current situation of the patient and should adapt to the patient's language.

The time frame in which is the no-suicide contract is valid, is individually negotiated with the patient and can range from several hours to several days. At each meeting in between and before the contract expires, the doctor assesses again the acute suicidality and negotiates a new contract with the patient. The result of the assessment may be recorded in the medical records or on the tab, e.g., the patient denies any current suicidal intent.

Practical Tip *Example of a written no-suicide contract/commitment-to-treatment-contract*

- If I am in danger, I will call.
- I will not kill myself intentionally or by carelessness, no matter what happens.
- I will not kill myself, no matter how I feel.
- I will use every opportunity that will help me in making decisions for continuing with my life.
- If I start to think about death, I will follow the emergency plan.
- I promise to do this until our next meeting.

Emergency Plan

The emergency plan serves the purpose of providing alternatives to suicide in the case of unbearable thoughts of suicide. It can be phrased as follows:

" In case of intolerable inner tensions and suicidal thoughts, I turn to . . . .

- My friend Erika
- My family doctor, Dr. Schmidt
- My psychotherapist, Dr. Franz
- To the emergency room of the psychiatric clinic
- To the telephone hot line

I find relief by telling my dialogue partner that I am in an unbearable state and I thought to commit suicide."

The emotional attachment to a reliable person is of vital importance for the prognosis. In addition to the persons close to them, this may be the doctor, of course.

After clarifying the whole situation and all outstanding issues, it must be discussed with the patient quite specifically, as to how things will continue on this very day and the time afterwards, who is available to support him/her, and how he/she will contact the doctor if the pressure inside increases again. The direct involvement in the conversation of, for example, family members or other trusted persons (if the patient agrees) and a tight scheduling of more appointments are valuable tools.

Pitfalls

- It is difficult to force activity from the patient that does not come from the patient himself, to at least some extent.
- Potential suicidality may be overlooked; that is why this has to be clarified at all times. It is not strange for depressive patients to be asked about suicidal thoughts; such questions do not amplify a potential suicidality either.
- The doctor wants to comfort and encourage the patient with the words: "Just think about how nice life can be . . . are you not thinking about your wife, your children? "Treat yourself to some 2 weeks vacation."
- The doctor actively takes measures without involving the patient (e.g., prescribing drugs, referral to a psychiatrist).
- The doctor is guided too much by the fear and panic of the patient and is no longer able to function.

Cooperation and Stepped Care

The treatment objective for depressive patients in a somatic-oriented setting is the initiation of a psychotherapeutical or psychopharmacological treatment. The physician should not go beyond giving information in the conversation. To work out subjacent conflicts or cognitive distortions that are associated with a depressive disorder requires a special training (Table 9.5).

In any case, the involvement of a psychiatric-psychotherapeutic specialist is required when a depressive symptomatology has reached moderate severity. The following treatment approaches alone or in combination may be considered: the cognitive behavioral therapy, psychoanalytically established procedures, and interpersonal therapy.

Cognitive behavior therapy, among other things, is about changing the acquired helplessness and cognitions and feelings of worthlessness, improving the emotional self-perception and the expression patterns, and promoting problem-solving strategies. This is achieved by methods such as the analysis of dysfunctional cognitions, testing reality by using the "Socratic dialogue" as well as the development of alternative cognitions.

The *psychoanalytic or psychodynamic therapy* aims at clarification, interpretation, and elaboration of conscious and unconscious interpersonal and intrapsychic conflicts. Here, early traumas and "object losses" are taken into account. Relationship patterns should be changed, conflicts managed. This is guided by the idea that the current situation of the patient is influenced by his/her past. The extent that this is individually significant will be experienced emotionally by the patient in the context of the therapeutic relationship.

Interpersonal therapy (*IPT*) has been developed specifically for the treatment of depressed patients. It is about the recognition of depression as an illness and the role of the patient as a sick person. The focus of treatment is on the relationship between depressive symptoms and current interpersonal stressors. IPT is a clearly structured treatment, the course of which is divided into three phases and should be completed in general after 16 sessions.

Cultural Aspects

Although depression could be seen as being universal according to the current mainstream theories, medical beliefs in different cultures influence the recognition, interpretation, and diagnosis of depression as well the help-seeking behavior of the patients remarkably. The core symptoms of depression, i.e., change of mood, disruption of physiological functions such as sleep and appetite, and hypochondriacal symptoms, are the same in Europe and in non-European cultures. Other symptoms such as feelings of guilt and suicidal tendencies showed variations of a frequency and intensity among cultures (Sartorius 1983).

In the WHO study (Simon et al. 1999), the somatic presentation of patients who met the criterion for Major Depression, was very different. A somatic presentation was more common at centers where patients lacked an ongoing relationship with a primary care physician than at centers where most patients had a personal physician.

Asia

A literature review published in the year 2001 confirmed an observation for decades that the Chinese people tend to deny depression and express it somatically (Parker et al. 2001). In Taiwan, social change, introduction of a universal national health insurance system and the effects of public education about depression increased the treatment rate of depression in the recent years (Chien et al. 2007).

Neither physicians of traditional Chinese medicine (TCM) diagnose depression nor do the patients who believe in TCM consider depressive mood on its own as an entity of medical disease in the sense of Western medicine. According to the classical theory of TCM, human being has seven essential emotions, i.e., happiness, anger, sorrow, concern, sadness, fear, fright. These emotions correspond with certain organs respectively (see introduction about TCM). If one of these emotions are imbalanced, e.g., it breaks the harmonious dynamic relations between Yin and Yang, between organs, etc., it could harm the organ it corresponds with (see chapter 4 about TCM). The TCM physicians see such a condition as a dynamic process instead of a constant status, which needs their continuous efforts to "re-balance" by prescribing herbal drugs. Of notice, is that the interpretation of diagnosis and prescription serves as a psychotherapeutic method for the patients, too.

In such a cultural context, most Chinese psychiatrists in 1980s preferred to diagnose depressive syndrome as neurasthenia. It became a new thing for them to see and to treat so many depressive patients just since 1990s. To some extent, this change can be understood as a result of the changes of conceptions about depression, not a substantial indicator that the Chinese are suffering much more from depression suddenly than before.

In Vietnam, the development of economics, changes in society and culture lead to change in living style, working environment, and population structure. These increased stress-related depression in the past decade. Depression in Vietnam is still stigmatized and under-recognized in community, family, and patient. The patient likes to see general doctors with lack of psychiatric knowledge, which delays the detection.

Symptoms of pain, eating disorders, etc. are often seen in depression, especially among elderly patients, menopaused women patients, etc. General doctors do not recognize the depressive symptoms and refer the patients to specialists, not psychiatrists. Loss of libido especially among Vietnamese women, are difficult to be aware and often ignored.

Medication is predominant in depression treatment. Application of psychotherapy is still limited in Vietnam. Superstitious methods are commonly used in remote and mountainous areas. Alcohol and substance abuse are applied as self treatment among patients.

Africa

Although as mentioned many symptoms are universal, local idioms are common, e.g., Kufungisisa in Shona in Zimbabwe. Some symptoms like loss of appetite may not be specific because of the abundant physical causes; some of the symptoms are culturally explained, e.g., seeing dead people in dreams calling the individual to join them. Causal attributions include relationship problems and supernatural causes. There is a complex relationship between depression, poverty, and economic deprivation (Fig. 9.4).

In African settings, treatment facilities are different in rural and urban areas and treatment is often dispensed in unconventional settings and may be combined with traditional methods (Patel et al. 2001).

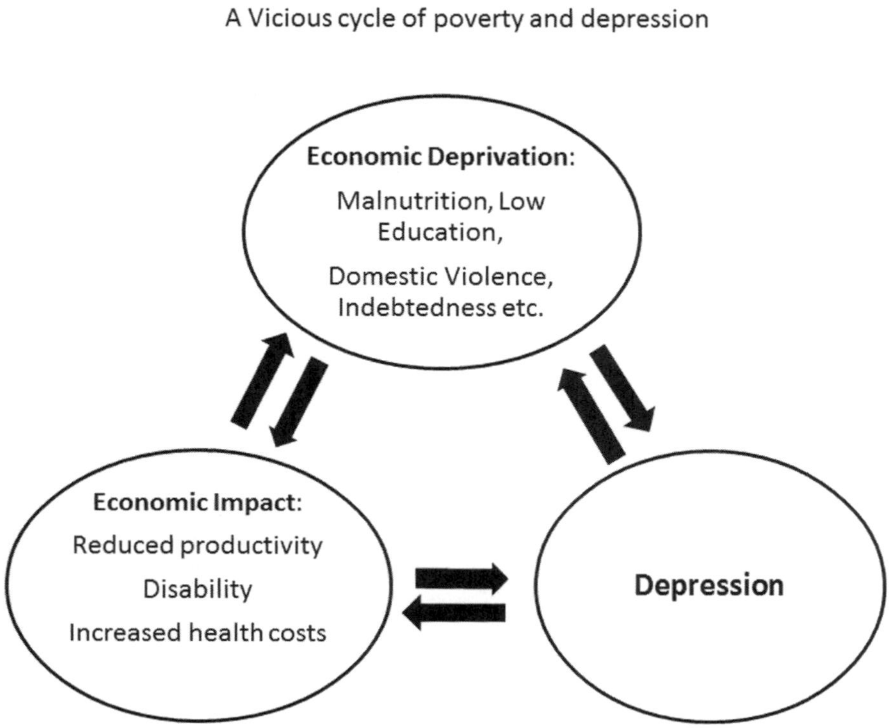

Fig. 9.4 Vicious cycle of poverty and depression

Latin America

Escobar et al. (1983) compared depressed inpatients in Colombia and USA. The results showed higher depression levels in Colombian patients. Raab and Mezzich (1980) compared depressed patients in Peru and USA. The incidence of endogenous depression was greater in the Peruvian sample. Associated factors in both countries were: Mestizo culture, lower educational level, to be female and married. This confirms the vicious cycle of poverty and depression shown in Fig. 9.4.

There is a high prevalence of postpartum depression (PPD) in the South of Brazil. Most acute cases and higher frequency are in general related to precarious economic conditions and lack of acceptance of pregnancy. This evidence puts pressure on public health authorities as regards to prevention and treatment, demanding integrated follow-up accounting for depression, measures such as home visits, at least to mothers with lower incomes are seen as crucial. It is important to emphasize, nonetheless, that poverty is considered one of the biggest villains for adequate care possibility.

Cultural Differences of Suicidal Behavior

The religious background and social attitudes decide whether to report on suicide. Many of the countries which are known for very low suicide rates include Muslim, Buddhist, or Catholic societies, where suicide is sanctioned by religious morality. Suicide rates are generally relatively stable for decades, however, sociocultural and political upheavals provide for changes. Motives for suicide vary across different societies. Suicidality in Eastern societies is closely related to mental or physical illness and associated adverse reactions for example, in the family. In undeveloped and developing countries, conflicts or financial problems are in the foreground. In Western societies, relationship problems or drug use play a larger role.

Family Suicide in Japan

The trigger is a socially intolerable situation for one or both parents such as financial debt or an incurable disease. Several reasons may cause the inclusion of children in family suicide: One reason is the fear that after the death of the parents no one will care for the children and that only parents can adequately care for them. Another reason is the strong family ties between parent and child: It is better to die as a family, than leaving behind a family member with a family that has been broken apart.

References

Arroll B, Khin N, Kerse N. Screening for depression in primary care with two verbally asked questions: cross sectional study. BMJ. 2003;327:1144–6.

Chien IC, Kuo CC, Bih SH, Chou YJ, Lin CH, Lee CH, Chou P. The prevalence and incidence of treated major depressive disorder among National Health Insurance Enrollees in Taiwan, 1996 to 2003. Can J Psychiatry. 2007;52(1):28–36.

Escobar JI, Gomez J, Tuason VB. Depressive symptomatology in North and South American patients. Am J Psychiatry. 1983;140(1):47–51.

Mezzich JE, Raab ES. Depressive symptomatology accross the Americas. Arch Gen Psychiatry. 1980;37(7):818–23.

Parker G, Gladstone G, Chee KT. Depression in the planet's largest ethnic group: the Chinese. Am J Psychiatry. 2001;158(6):857–64.

Patel V, Abas M, Broadhead J, Todd C, Reeler A. Depression in developing countries: lessons from Zimbabwe. BMJ. 2001;322:482.

Sartorius N, Davidian H, Ernberg G, Fenton FR, Jujii I, Gastpar M. Depressive disorders in different cultures: report on the WHO collaborative study on standardized assessment of depressive disorders. World Health Organization; 1983.

Simon GE, von Korff M, Piccinelli M, Fullerton C, Ormel J. An international study of the relation between somatic symptoms and depression. New Engl J Med. 1999;341(18):1329–35.

Wittchen HU, Jacobi F, Rehm J, Gustavsson A, Svensson M, Jönsson B, et al. The size and burden of mental disorders and other disorders of the brain in Europe 2010. Eur Neuropsychopharm. 2011;21:655–79.

Chapter 10
Anxiety Disorders

Kurt Fritzsche

Case Study "Agoraphobia" A 41-year-old female patient developed blurred vision and very unpleasant and rather unspecific dizziness after an acute flu-like infection. She was on sick leave for a fairly long period because of these debilitating symptoms, several attempts to become accustomed to a new job as a legal secretary failed. In particular, she was unable to tolerate working with the computer monitor. A few months before, she had lost the job she had for years, because her boss gave up his law practice. Consequently, she has withdrawn more and more, leaves the house increasingly infrequently and does not dare driving the car, since she caused a slight dent when parking in the garage. Since she lives in the countryside, this vastly limits her mobility.

(continued)

Definition

Anxiety is one of the basic human experiences. Patterns of anxiety accompany all emotional and physical illnesses, either openly or disguised. The disposition to feel fear guarantees individual survival, similar to the capability of feeling pain. To have no fear at all may be just as unusual or remarkable as having too much fear.

Fear is useful and necessary as:

- Alarm signal in response to threatening events
- Preparation of the body to act quickly
- Standby mode for escape and avoidance

Fear becomes an illness when:

- It is unreasonably strong
- It occurs too often and for too long

K. Fritzsche (✉)
Department of Psychosomatic Medicine and Psychotherapy, University Medical Center, Hauptstr. 8, 79104 Freiburg, Germany
e-mail: kurt.fritzsche@uniklinik-freiburg.de

K. Fritzsche et al. (eds.), *Psychosomatic Medicine*, DOI 10.1007/978-1-4614-1022-5_10,

Table 10.1 Anxiety symptoms on four levels

Behaviour	Feelings	Body	Thoughts
Avoidance, flight	Feelings of tension, worry, panic, unreality, fear of going crazy, of dying, of losing control	Trembling, sweating, heart pounding, light-headedness, dizziness, muscle tension, nausea, breathlessness, numbness, stomach pains, tingling sensation	Something terrible is going to happen, I have got to get out of here, I am despairing

- One loses control over it
- One must avoid anxiety situations
- It leads to restriction of daily life
- It leads to abuse of alcohol or drugs and
- One severely suffers from it

Anxiety involves complex physical and emotional simultaneous episodes, which are reflected on four levels (Table 10.1).

Relevance

In anxiety disorders often physical symptoms, as so-called affective equivalents, are in place of consciously perceived fear. This aspect is particularly important in psychosomatic primary care, since patients experiencing physical symptoms primarily turn to their GP or a specialist, if necessary. Anxiety disorders are often not diagnosed, misdiagnosed or diagnosed too late, and are rarely treated specifically and appropriately. Untreated, anxiety disorders usually run a chronic course and spontaneous remissions are rare. There are high comorbidities with other mental disorders such as depression and somatoform disorders. All this suggests that timely detection saves huge costs in primary care.

Theory

Symptoms

In a large number of patients with anxiety disorder, feelings are hidden behind physical symptoms. Table 10.2 shows an overview of physical symptoms of anxiety, arranged by organ systems.

Table 10.2 Physical symptoms of fear

Heart	Irregular, rapid or pounding heartbeat to palpitations, left-thoracic sensation of pressure
Vascular system	Pallor or flush in the face and extremities, cold-sweaty hands and feet, hypertension
Musculature	Tremors, weak knees, motor restlessness, muscle tension, feeling of paralysis, pain in the joints, arms and legs, tingling and numbness
Respiratory tract	Hyperventilation, feeling of constriction and shortness of breath, fear of suffocation
Gastrointestinal tract	Lump in the throat (Globus) with difficulty swallowing, swallowing air and belching, vomiting, stomach ache, diarrhoea
Vegetative/autonomic nervous system	Sweating, dilated pupils, need to urinate
Central nervous system	Dizziness and giddiness, tremors, spots before the eyes, impaired vision, such as double vision, headache, insomnia, impaired concentration, fatigue, weakness, depersonalisation and derealisation

Diagnostic Categories

Panic Disorder (ICD 10 F 40.01)

The most essential characteristics are recurrent phases of intensive acute fear, so-called panic attacks. They do not refer to a certain situation and are experienced by the patient usually as spontaneously occurring palpitations, chest pain, feeling of suffocation, severe dizziness, headache, up to a feeling of alienation. In addition, fear of dying or going mad does occur. These occur spontaneously, are completely unexpected, and last from a few minutes to an hour.

Case Study: "Panic disorder" A 36-year-old patient, mother of three sons, developed severe panic attacks, which completely undermined her stability, after her husband changed his behaviour—for her unexpectedly and inconceivably. He dyed his hair and announced that from then on, he was going to do his own thing and do as he pleased. In the preceding years, at high personal cost, the two had renovated the house they had taken over from the parents.

The patient felt completely overwhelmed, helpless and unable to act and hardly able to cope with the daily tasks of keeping the house. She was repeatedly overcome by great feelings of fear, coupled with palpitations, severe dizziness, sweating and trembling. Often she felt herself on the border of "losing control" or "flipping out", so her husband sometimes thought she might jump off the balcony under the pressure of the situation.

She was able, little by little, to cope better with her fears, bear unpleasant states of tension and become able to conduct her life only after intensive long-term psychotherapy, several months of in-hospital treatment in a special clinic and a temporary use of anxiolytics and antidepressives.

A deep underlying rift in the marital relationship was identified which had long been building up under the surface. The two finally decided to separate.

Phobic Anxiety Disorders (F40)

Agoraphobia (ICD-10: F 40.00 Without Panic Attacks, F40.01 with Panic Attacks)

Many patients with panic attacks come to avoid places in which anxiety attacks occurred. The avoidance behaviour may reach a stage in which many patients are unable to leave their house. Agoraphobia describes not only the fear of open places, but also, for example, of crowds, or the desire to be able to leave on the spot and to retreat easily to a safe place. Typical situations which these patients avoid or endure only with severe anxiety include department stores, cinemas, restaurants, public transportation, driving a car, lifts or heights. Most patients report they can endure the feared situation better in company. As a substitute for a fear-reducing trusted person, the patient may take along medications, smelling substances or the doctor's telephone number. Agoraphobia may also develop without any preceding acute anxiety attack or panic attacks. These patients often report a rather diffuse feeling of eeriness and threat which comes over them when they leave their familiar environment.

Case Study: "Agoraphobia" (continued) Numerous specialist examinations and hospital treatment follow to definitely rule out any possibly organic cause of the illness. She does not tolerate antidepressive medications. A 2-month rehabilitation programme in hospital and outpatient group psychotherapy is needed to enable her to work at least part time and to cope with everyday life without more significant limitations.

Social phobias (ICD-10: F 40.1)

Predominant is an inappropriate fear and avoidance of situations in which the patient has to deal with other people and may be judged. They are afraid of failure, being laughed at or being belittled because of clumsy behaviour. A social phobia may be limited to specific situations, such as eating or speaking in public, or meeting someone they do not know very well. The patients express complaints as blushing, trembling hands, nausea or the urge to urinate.

Case Study: "Social Phobia" A 25-year-old medical student has increasing problems eating in the company of others, in the cafeteria, for example. He has the feeling he cannot swallow a bite or suffers from a severe, almost irresistible urge to gag. With time, he avoids such situations, which means he is often alone, can concentrate entirely on his studies, but sometimes is so restless that the eating problem even occurs at home, though in a weaker form. It is found that he often felt insecure in dealing with others, and even before, he thought he was too fat, sweats too much and would make others uncomfortable by his presence.

Although he is studying nearly 750 km away from home, he is in very close contact with his family and is often asked for advice by his father, for instance. His father is very proud of him because he is the first one in the whole family to attend university.

The patient's problem is a separation problem from the parental home. His need for autonomy surfaces only indirectly. When he receives the news that after his exams next year he can participate in a research project in the USA, he is able to eat an entire meal at McDonald's with no problem. In this situation, he does not experience any symptoms any more.

Specific (isolated) Phobias (ICD-10: F 40.2)

Here, the fear is limited to the proximity to certain animals, heights, thunder, darkness, flying, the sight of blood, injuries or the fear of being exposed to certain diseases, such as AIDS. The extent of the disorder depends on how easily the patient can avoid the phobic situation or the phobic object.

Generalised Anxiety Disorder (ICD-10 F 41.1)

Typical are generalised and persistent fears, which are not, however, limited to certain situations in the environment. They refer to fears and worries in several areas of life, such as workplace, partnership etc.

Case Study: "Generalised anxiety disorder" A 38-year-old patient reacts to a change in his job, which for him is completely unexpected when his boss retires, with very severe anxiety and deep helpless despair. He feels incapable of resisting these feelings, experiences to be passively doomed, like falling into a chasm. Only intensive psychiatric-psychotherapeutic support can very gradually give him more stability.

After he tried—from his perspective in vain—for several months to get along with the new boss, by reducing his working time, for example, he decides to resign, which throws him into a new crisis after an extremely short phase of relief. Again, his situation does not stabilise for several months, until he has the opportunity to enter an extensive training programme offered by the state employment office.

It is discovered that he has suffered severe fear of illness, permanent lack of self-confidence and considerable trouble in making decisions since his childhood, which were interrupted for only brief periods by phases of greater stability.

Hypochondriacal Disorder (ICD-10: F 45.2)

The patient is constantly concerned with the possibility of having one or more serious and progressive physical diseases. General physical sensations are interpreted as abnormal and stressful and ascribed to a serious disease.

Somatoform Autonomic Dysfunction of the Heart and Cardiovascular System (ICD-10: F 45.3)

In this discrete phobia, the feared object is not part of the external world, but part of one's own body. The focus is fear of an unrecognised heart disease and the fear of dying a cardiac death. The symptoms often correspond to those of angina pectoris, but are demonstratively dwelt upon. Heart phobics do not have an elevated risk of heart attack. But by continually undergoing examination, despite unremarkable findings, the patient's conviction that he is suffering from a serious disease becomes stronger.

Obsessive–Compulsive Disorder (ICD-10: F42)

The core features of these disorders are obsessions (intrusive, unwanted thoughts) and compulsions (performance of highly ritualised behaviours intended to neutralise the negative thoughts and emotions resulting from the obsessions). One symptom pattern might be repetitive hand washing beyond the point of skin damage to neutralise fears of contamination.

Differential Diagnosis

The following important somatic differential diagnoses must be taken into consideration:

- Hyperthyroidism
- Coronary heart disease
- Paroxysmal tachycardia
- Pheochromocytoma
- Hypoglycaemia
- Cerebral seizures
- Drug side effects
- Drug abuse

Frequency and Course

Anxiety disorders have a lifetime prevalence of 14 % in European countries, making them the most common emotional disorders among the general public. The following lifetime prevalence rates are found for individual anxiety disorders: specific phobia 6.4 %, social phobia 2.3 %, agoraphobia, 2 %, panic disorder 1.8 % and generalised anxiety disorder, 1.7 % (young people) to 3.4 % (elderly) (Wittchen et. al. 2011).

There is a risk of chronicity mainly in secondary abuse of alcohol and/or medication, comorbid depression and an excessive number of visits of the medical and psychosocial institutions.

Onset

The following three factors of the biopsychosocial model play a varying role in patients suffering from an anxiety disorder:

Neurobiological Changes

Congenital and acquired elevated neurophysiological excitability accompanied by feelings of anxiety are stored in the amygdala and hippocampus. This emotional memory is long term, can be activated in certain situations, but also inhibited via controlling impulses from the prefrontal cortex by psychotherapeutic and psychopharmacological means. Moreover, there is a dysfunction of serotonin and noradrenalin metabolism in anxiety patients.

Psychosocial Disposition

Coping with fear is one of the developmental tasks set for every human in passing through the various phases of life. If the parents' childrearing style is not very empathic and offers little protection or overprotecting, this is detrimental to strengthening mechanisms for coping with fear in conflict situations. Elicitors of anxious states are typical threshold situations like puberty, end of the school years, leaving the parental home, marriage, when children leave home, end of professional life or death of someone close, for example. A reliable bond constitutes a good protection against the onset of an anxiety disorder.

Stressful Life Events and Illness

These events include changes in habitual circumstances, e.g. moving to another city or a different country, the real or expected loss of someone close, situation at the job or at home. Fear of death occurs with the feeling of suffocation in an acute attack of bronchial asthma or heart attack.

Practice

Recognition

Example of an Introduction "Many people are frightened in a wide variety of situations. Can you tell me if the following situations or things would frighten you or make you want to avoid them?"

Sample of Anamnesis Questions

Panic Syndrome "Do you sometimes suffer from sudden and unexpected panic attacks, even though there is no real threat?"

Agoraphobia "Are there certain situations or places, like department stores, driving a car, crowds of people, lifts or closed rooms, that frighten you or that you avoid wherever possible?"

Social Phobia "Are you frightened by or do you avoid certain situations in which you might be observed or judged by other people, such as speaking in public, eating, parties etc.?"

Specific Phobia Do certain things or activities frighten you, such as animals, heights, flying, the sight of blood or injuries?"

Generalised Anxiety Syndrome "Do you often suffer from excessive worries that you cannot control, such as family matters, your job or finances?"

Obsessive-Compulsive Syndrome "Are there senseless or unpleasant thoughts or acts that you cannot get out of your mind, or which you have to do over and over, even though you try to stop?"

Basic Therapeutic Attitude

Patients with anxiety disorders are friendly, adapted and happy to have found a doctor in whom they have confidence and who treats them well. At the same time, however, they tend to distancelessly cling to and use the doctor as a person who gives them security, without any consideration of him/her or his/her interests. An ideal posture for treatment is avoidance of overprotectiveness without abandoning the patient or overtaxing him. The doctor endures the patient's contact hunger and need for security, is not upset by the many complaints but gives the impression of both constancy and safety.

You can structure a helpless regressive patient by permitting him choices and thus strengthening his capacity for action and decision. It is possible to list a number of problem areas and to ask the patient to decide on their order of importance and the sequence in which they should be treated. An example would be, "We now have three topics: topic one, topic two, topic three. What would you like to talk about first? What second and what third? I'll make a note of the order."

Basic Interventions

Strengthening Autonomy

The patient's self-responsibility and self-confidence should be maintained, protected and also promoted. In cooperation with the patient, the doctor attempts to find out

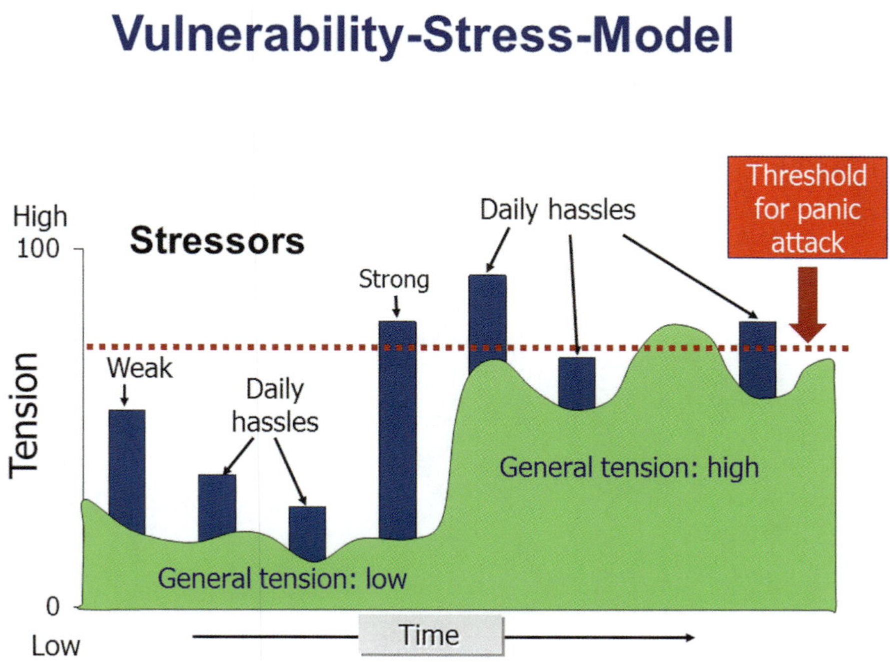

Fig. 10.1 Stress vulnerability

what the patient feels, what he/she can do despite his/her complaints and limitations and what recommendations and suggestions he/she can put into practice. Changes occur usually only in small steps. Relapses are to be expected if too great steps lead to overtaxing. In developing countries where the doctor is viewed as the person who has the power to heal, statements like "Doctor, you are the one who knows what I must do in order to get well" should be counteracted gently.

Psychoeducation

As shown schematically in Fig. 10.1, for each patient suffering from anxiety, the physical and mental stress level is increased dramatically:

> Doctor: When there is too much tension our body often reacts with feelings of anxiety and stress symptoms (rapid heartbeat, shortness of breath, sweaty palms . . .). In generally low internal tension, it usually takes a long time until it comes to anxiety reactions. If your inner tension is very high, even just a little bit of stress can be the straw to break the camel's back.

Relaxation Techniques

A first general measure involves reducing the increased internal tension through a relaxation technique such as progressive muscle relaxation according to Jacobsen. This achieves a significant anxiety reduction.

Fig. 10.2 Vicious circle of fear

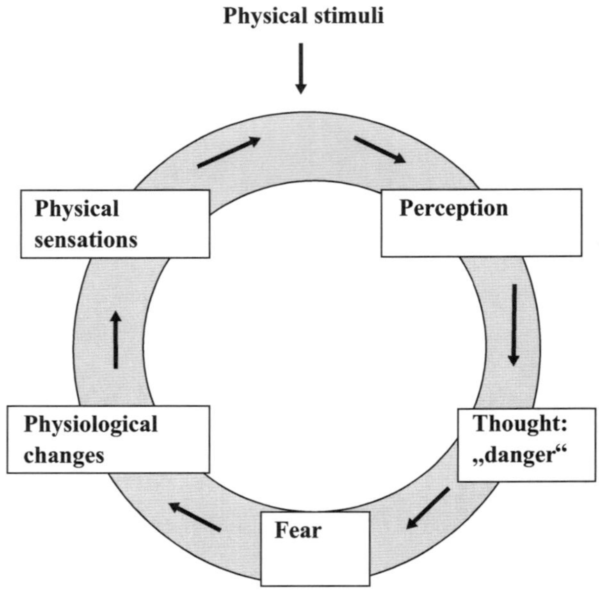

The Vicious Circle of Fear

The onset and maintenance of an anxiety disorder can best be explained to the patient as a "vicious circle". In people who tend to particularly strong physical vegetative reactions or those who observe themselves especially intensively, fear may lead to perceiving only the physical changes but not the accompanying emotional factors. Such people tend to work themselves into a state of "fear of the fear", whereby the pressure of expectation and tension itself results in eliciting fear signals. This process can become stronger and stronger in the vicious circle, leaving the patient feeling completely at the mercy of events (Fig. 10.2).

Practical tip: Examples of Breaking the Vicious Circle: "Exposure" and "Cognitive Restructuring" The patient experiences shortness of breath and palpitations as a threat and thinks: "Soon I have to die". To correct the misperception and misinterpretation of his/her physical symptoms, the patient is instructed to develop a new fear reducing assessment of physical symptoms. In addition, he/she will get used to these complaints by specific confrontation with the anxiety-provoking symptoms and will experience them to be harmless. Suitable for this confrontation are, e.g. squats, walking in place, jump rope, sauna and gym for the generation of heart palpitations and sweating.

In patients with anxiety-related functional respiratory disorders, which often lead to hyperventilation conditions, the symptoms may be caused directly by a joint exercise wherein in the office the patient is forced to inhale and exhale until the first physical symptoms such as tightness, mild dizziness or tingling sensation under the skin occur by doing so, the patient experiences the harmlessness of his/her complaints and

Table 10.3 Drug treatment in anxiety disorders

Benzodiazepines	Phytotherapeutic substances	Antidepressives
Brief efficacy confirmed in panic attacks (esp. Alprazolam); problems of dependency and tolerance	Used in general anxiety and increased susceptibility to anxiety, evidence is lacking	SSRIs, SSNRIs proven for panic disorders and social phobia; in generalised anxiety disorder sometimes effective even in low doses

that he himself/she herself has control over them. In severe hyperventilation, the CO_2 rebreathing in a plastic bag or cupped hands that surround the nose can be performed.

Drug Treatment

Patients with anxiety disorders are often sceptical about treatment with medications and fear side effects or becoming addicted. For this reason, it is important to discuss the effects and side effects of the medication in detail with the patient and to take his/her subjective reactions absolutely seriously. If a person with anxiety disorder chooses drug treatment, offer a selective serotonin reuptake inhibitor (SSRI). Monitor the person carefully for adverse reactions (Table 10.3).

Taking into account the following factors:

- Tendency to experience withdrawal symptoms (especially with paroxetine and venlafaxine)
- Side-effect profile and potential for drug–drug interactions
- The risk of suicide and likelihood of toxicity in case of overdose (especially with venlafaxine)
- The person's prior experience of treatment with particular drugs (particularly adherence, effectiveness, side effects, experience of withdrawal symptoms and the person's preference).

Do not offer a benzodiazepine except as a short-term measure during crises. Do not offer an antipsychotic for the treatment!

Crisis Intervention in Panic Attack

If a person presents with a panic attack, he/she should be asked if they are already receiving treatment for panic disorder. It should be undergone the minimum examination necessary to exclude acute physical problems. The patients should be given appropriate written information about panic attacks, about sources of support (Table 10.4).

In panic attacks, it is necessary to calm the patient. Speak in a calm, confident and friendly voice. Try to normalise the physical sensations of the patient. At the same time, strengthen his/her reality testing and make it clear that he/she has no reason to

Table 10.4 Written information about panic attacks for patients

Even anxious patients have no greater risk that a feared catastrophe might occur than any other people
Unpleasant feelings belong to the emotional world of every person. So do not waste energy unnecessarily trying to suppress fear, since this cannot be successful in the long term
Overcoming fear is most successful if you are willing to admit unpleasant feelings, to stay in the situation without giving up until the fear abates
When you practice facing fearful situations, the following attitudes and sentences can help you:
It is all right to be afraid
I will see this situation through
The physical symptoms certainly will not last
I will feel relieved and stronger when it is over
The concurrent physical symptoms in a fearful situation are very unpleasant, but they are neither damaging nor dangerous. The goal of your exercise is to learn to deal with fear and not to avoid it
Learn where your personal stress limits are and try to stay within those limits, since too much physical-emotional stress is often the basis for anxiety disorders

be frightened. Positive suggestive measures may be helpful. For example, you could symbolically feel his/her pulse.

Practical Tip "What you are now experiencing is a panic attack. Your heart is beating faster; you have trouble breathing. I can understand that this upsets you. You feel as though you are in great danger. I want to tell you that there is nothing to be afraid of. Here in my room, you are completely safe and your heart is physically healthy. Nothing is going to happen to you. I will stay with you until the attack is over. I can already see that your heart is beating more slowly and calmly now."

Practical Tip: "Techniques of Panic Management"

- Use of breathing techniques
- Focus attention, e.g. "Tell me five things that you see right now."
- "Reality check" of irrational beliefs
- Supportive self-instructions with simultaneous perception of physical signals

Especially if the patient is worried about "going mad" or being incurably ill, it may be helpful if you do not stress the pathological, but rather the underlying normality of the experience and behaviour, from which the patient has gradually deviated.

Practical Tip "Actually, it's quite normal that you are worried. But we should ask ourselves why your worry has become so strong that you are completely anxious.

I believe anybody would have been annoyed in such a situation. But your annoyance was stronger than that; you became completely irate."

Pitfalls

- The confident, motherly caring doctor tries to provide a fearful patient with maternal security, protection and warmth. For a brief period of time, the doctor and

Table 10.5 Stepped care model of treatment in anxiety disorders

GP consultation and education
The use of relaxation techniques
Use of herbal preparations
Recommendation of a self-help group
Short-term administration of psychotropic drugs
Psychiatric consultation with/without psychotherapy
Combination treatment psychotherapy/psychotropics
Inpatient treatment

the patient are comfortable in this constellation. In the long term, however, this doctor may cause harm to the patient in that the overprotective attitude may inhibit his/her chances for an emancipatory development.

- An insecure doctor with depressive personality will try to get rid of a patient suffering from an anxiety disorder. The clinging behaviour and the repetitive requests for reassurance or for medical examination are a nuisance and can lead to impatience and anger. The insecure doctor avoids to empathise with the helplessness of the patient. He/she provides little support to the patient and tries to get rid of him/her by advice that seems overwhelming to the patient.

It is important that the doctor as a helper keeps the necessary distance. There is a high risk that he/she too heavily identifies with the patient or even becomes infected by his/her fear. In the worst case it could lead to unnecessary therapeutic activism obscuring the problem rather than clarifying it.

Cooperation and Stepped Care (Table 10.5)

Good evidence exists that both drug and psychosocial treatments are effective in managing anxiety disorders (NICE guidelines 2011).

Severe and complex forms of anxiety disorders require professional psychotherapeutic treatment. If the management of anxiety symptoms is in the foreground, a cognitive *behavioural* therapy is indicated. Treatment programs usually contain components that have been mentioned earlier in the basic therapy, and which are now used in a more targeted and more intense manner: providing information about anxiety and panic attacks, distorted perception and interpretation of physical symptoms originally interpreted as threatening and the confrontation with anxiety-provoking thoughts when anxiety symptoms occur.

If by contrast the detection and processing of unconscious conflicts is indicated, *psychoanalytically founded therapies* are preferred. Primarily, these procedures are not symptom oriented, rather they are personality oriented.

Cultural Aspects

The cultural background has a significant effect on the expression of fear.

People in different cultures express their emotions in different ways in language, gestures and physical reactions and facial expressions. In most cases, both physical symptoms and psychological symptoms of anxiety are present. Also, many everyday phrases (idioms) show the relationship between emotions and body such as, for example, "Butterflies in the stomach" or "a pain in the neck". In Chinese, there are expressions like "lost spleen spirit"—meaning loosing ones temper or "elevated liver fire", meaning being emotionally aroused (Kirmayer and Young 1998; Tseng 2006; Karasz et al. 2007).

In Asian countries, for example, people tend to inhibit expressing their anxiety due to beliefs of the traditional Chinese medicine and the folk religion, a mixture of Confucianism, Taoism, Buddhism and shamanism. Patients with anxiety disorders and their family may seek help from doctors of traditional medicine and from religious healers in temples rather than from psychiatric services (Ma et al. 2010).

Some examples of culture-specific manifestations of fear are presented below.

Tai-jin-kyofu-sho (Japan)

Tai-jin-kyofu-sho means disorder of fear of interpersonal relations or "anthrophobia" in contrast to patients with social phobia, which have a marked persistent fear of social performance situation in which the person is exposed to unfamiliar people. Patients with *tai-jin-kyofu-sho* are more concerned with self in other's view, associated with feelings of embarrassment and many dismorphobic concerns. They are eager to socialise with others and have no problems relating with strangers, but are concerned with how to properly relate to friends, colleagues or superiors. The same difficulties with a familiar group in semiprivate circumstances are found in Korea, but not in China (Kitanesh et al. 1995).

Dhat Syndrome (Asia)

Patients, mostly young men, often present multiple somatic symptoms such as fatigue, weakness, anxiety or feelings of guilt, supposedly caused by loss of semen such as masturbation or prostitution. In India, it is referred to as *Dhat* syndrome, in Sri Lanka, Nepal, Bangladesh and Pakistan as *Pramha*, and in Taiwan as *Shenkui*. The common belief is that the loss of semen can lead to disease.

Koro (China)

First described in 1934 in southern China, and later in other parts of Asia and Africa. The fear of a sudden disappearance of sex organs (penis, but also breast), usually by retracting into the body.

Frigophobia (China)

Frigophobia is a morbid fear of catching a cold. It develops because of an imbalance between Yin and Yang. Excessive Yin caused by cold air or excessive eating of cold food will result in weakness and sickness.

Heart Distress (Iran)

"Heart distress" is seen as a manifestation of anxiety and depressive disorders (Good and Good 1982). It ranges from mild excitations to fainting and heart attack. (See also chapter about coronary heart disease).

Susto (Latin America)

Susto ("Soul loss syndrome") is widespread in Latin America. It is based on the idea that the body and soul are two separable components of the human being. The soul leaves the body when a spirit steals it. According to statements by the people, "susto" occurs mainly in children because their soul is weaker. Physical symptoms are: loss of appetite, nausea, vomiting and diarrhoea. The children are scared, scream and cry particularly at night. Many symptoms of "susto" are treated with herbs. There are also other forms of magic treatment "calling the soul" through a traditional healer who prays to benign spirits in order to recover the soul.

References

Good BJ, Good MJD. Toward a meaning- centered analysis of popular illness categories: "Fright Illness" and "Heart Distress" in Iran. In: Marsella AJ, White GM, editor. Cultural conceptions of mental health and illness. D. Reidel publishing company; 1982:141–66.

Karasz A, Dempsey K, Fallek R. Cultural differences in the experiences of everyday symptoms: a comparative study of South Asian and European American women. Cult Med Psychiatry. 2007;31(4):473–97.

Kirmayer LJ, Young A. Culture and somatization: clinical, epidemiological and ethnographic perspectives. Psychosom Med. 1998;60(4):420–30.

Kitanish K, Miyake Y, Kim KI, Liu XH. A comparative study of taijinkyofusho (TSK) tendencies among college students in Japan, Korea and the People's Republic of China. Jikeikai Med J. 1995;42(3):231–43.

Ma WF, Huang XY, Chang HJ, Yen WJ, Lee S. Impact of Taiwanese culture on beliefs about expressing anxiety and engaging in physical activity: a discursive analysis of the literature. J Clin Nursing. 2010;19:969–77.

NICE. Generalised anxiety disorder and panic disorder—clinical guidelines. http://www.nice.org.uk/nicemedia/Live/13314/52601/52601.pdf.

Tseng WS. From peculiar psychiatric disorders through culture-bound syndromes to culture-related specific syndromes. Transcult Psychiatry 2006;43(4):554–76.

Wittchen HU, Jacobi F, Rehm J, Gustavsson A, Svensson M, Jönsson B, et al. The size and burden of mental disorders and other disorders of the brain in Europe 2010. Eur Neuropsychopharmacol. 2011;21:655–79.

Chapter 11
Somatoform Disorders

Kurt Fritzsche, Kim Viet Nguyen, Van Tuan Nguyen, Catherine Abbo, Gertrud Frahm, Sonia Diaz Monsalve, Lan Zhang and Jing Wei

Case Study Since childhood, Mrs. D. has regularly suffered from lower abdominal pain, sometimes associated with frequent bowel movements. She has not seen a doctor for the complaints for a long time. She has become accustomed to the on and off pain. For several weeks, the symptoms do not disappear completely. The pain has also worsened; it is so bad at times that she cannot fall asleep at night. She wakes up at night and has to go urgently to the toilet again and again, and this tenesmus is the worst for her. If it comes, she must immediately go to the toilet because she is afraid she cannot hold her stool, and

K. Fritzsche (✉) · S. D. Monsalve
Department of Psychosomatic Medicine and Psychotherapy,
University Medical Center, Hauptstr. 8, 79104 Freiburg, Germany
e-mail: kurt.fritzsche@uniklinik-freiburg.de

S. D. Monsalve
e-mail: sonia.diaz-monsalve@uniklinik-freiburg.de

K. V. Nguyen · V. T. Nguyen
Department of Psychiatry, Hanoi Medical University, No. 1, Ton That Tung Street, Dong Da District, Hanoi, Vietnam
e-mail: drnkimviet@yahoo.com

National Institute of Mental Health, Bach Mai Hospital, No. 78, Giai Phong Road, Dong Da District, Hanoi, Vietnam

V. T. Nguyen
e-mail: nvtuannimhvn@hmu.edu.vn

C. Abbo
Department of Psychiatry, Makerere University College of Health Sciences and Mulago National Referral and Teaching Hospital, Mulago Hill Road, P.O. Box 7072, Kampala, Uganda
e-mail: cathyabbo@chs.mak.ac.ug, cathya180@gmail.com

G. Frahm
Department of Human Sciences, Federal University of Paraná,
R. Gal. Carneiro, 460, Curitiba, PR 80060-150, Brazil
e-mail: gfrahm@uol.com.br

K. Fritzsche et al. (eds.), *Psychosomatic Medicine,* DOI 10.1007/978-1-4614-1022-5_11,

the pressure is also very painful. Since she works by the hour as an assistant in a clothing store, she is very embarrassed. She always thinks of new excuses to tell to clients and colleagues, however, she herself no longer thinks of those excuses as being credible.
(continued)

Definition

Internationally, the terms 'Medically Unexplained Symptoms' (MUS), 'functional somatic syndromes' and the diagnostic category 'somatoform disorders' of classification systems DSM and ICD are currently being used. MUS and 'functional somatic syndromes' are broader terms and do not carry a risk of stigmatisation of the patient. Especially in primary care settings in Western countries, the term 'medically unexplained symptoms' has gained popularity in recent years to describe the bodily complaints of patients when the aetiology is unclear.

The following terms may be distinguished:

a. *Medically unexplained symptoms (MUS)*: general term, very broad
b. *Functional syndromes*: disturbance of bodily function rather than structure
c. *Somatization*: a psychological problem or emotional disorder is expressed somatically
d. *Somatoform disorders*: Diagnostic category in the psychiatric classification of Diagnostic and Statistical Manual of Mental Disorders (DSM) and International Classification of Diseases (ICD)

According to ICD 10, a somatoform disorder is characterized by the following features:

- Repeated presentation of somatic symptoms
- Stubborn and persistent demand for medical examination despite negative organic findings (dysfunctional illness behaviour)
- Emotional problems denied, although there is close relationship with psychosocial life events or conflicts (somatic fixation)
- Disappointing doctor–patient relationship (interpersonal disorder)

L. Zhang
Department of Psychiatry, West China Hospital, No. 37 Guoxue Lane, Chengdu 610041, Sichuan, P.R. China
e-mail: lanzhang3@gmail.com

J. Wei
Department of Psychological Medicine, Peking Union Medical College Hospital, 1 Shuaifuyuan, Dongcheng District, 100730 Beijing, P. R. China
e-mail: weijing@pumch.cn

Table 11.1 Manifestations of somatoform symptoms

Organ system	Frequent symptoms
Heart	Chest pains, paroxysmal tachycardias
Blood pressure	Hypertension and hypotension regulation disorders, syncope
Upper gastrointestinal tract	Nausea, feeling of repletion, meteorism
Lower gastrointestinal tract	Pain, diarrhoea, obstipation
Respiration	Hyperventilation with paresthesias
Motor apparatus	Back pain
Urogenital system	Urination problems, menstruation problems
Nervous system	Dizziness, convulsions, paralysis
General symptoms	Reduced performance capacity, insomnias

Relevance

About 20 % of patients who consult the family doctor have physical complaints with no adequate organic finding. The treatment of patients with symptoms without medical diagnosis is difficult. The patients explain their symptoms through a previously unrecognized physical illness, and initially, do not accept psychosomatic explanations. Because of the ensuing, often poorly developed motivation for psychotherapy, these patients are treated more frequently in general hospitals and medical practices of different disciplines than by a specialist in outpatient or inpatient psychotherapy. Extended time on disability and high costs due to the extensive use of inadequate medical diagnostics in outpatient and inpatient care when symptoms persist, demonstrate the importance of somatization phenomena in health care.

Theory

Symptoms

Somatoform symptoms may affect any organ system. The most frequent manifestations are shown in Table 11.1.

Most of the complaints listed in Table 11.1 are ascribed to certain diagnoses. It is thus suggested that the disease is physical. Accordingly, therapeutic success with medication, operation and other primarily somatic-oriented therapeutic procedures is low. Table 11.2 presents an overview of the diagnoses found in a wide variety of specialties, and in which somatization is usually present.

Table 11.2 Diagnosis in various specialties

Speciality	Diagnoses
Allergology	Allergy to foods
Cardiology	Non-cardiac chest pains
	Mitral valve prolapse
Dentistry	Complaints with mandibular joint
	Atypical facial pain
General practice	Tinnitus
	Dizziness
	Globus syndrome
Gynaecology	Premenstrual syndrome
	Chronic lower abdominal pain
Occupational medicine	Multiple chemical sensitivity (MCS)
	Chronic fatigue syndrome (CFS)
	Sick building syndrome[a]
Orthopaedics	Prolapsed disc
Pneumology	Dyspnea
	Hyperventilation
Rehabilitation medicine	Whiplash
Rheumatology	Fibromyalgia
Military medicine	Gulf War syndrome[b]

[a]Unspecific symptoms like headache, nausea and rash on staying in buildings for longer periods
[b]Marked fatigue, skin rash, impaired sense of smell etc. in English and American soldiers who participated in the 1990 Gulf War

Diagnostic Categories

Somatoform Disorders (ICD-10: F 45)

The following subclassification has proven helpful in practice :

- *Undifferentiated somatoform disorder* (ICD-10: F 45.1): Multiple somatoform symptoms for at least 6 months.
- *Somatoform autonomic dysfunction* of the vegetatively supplied organ systems like the heart, gastrointestinal tract, respiration and urogenital system (ICD-10: F 45.3) (Table 11.1).
- Persistent somatoform *pain disorders* (ICD-10: F 45.4)
- *Hypochondriacal disorders* (ICD-10: F 45.2): The patient is excessively occupied over long periods with the possibility of suffering from one or more serious, progressive physical diseases. Everyday physical sensations are misinterpreted as threatening and stressful.
- In *body dysmorphic disorders,* the body is interpreted as being deformed. This is usually accompanied by a desire for cosmetic surgery.

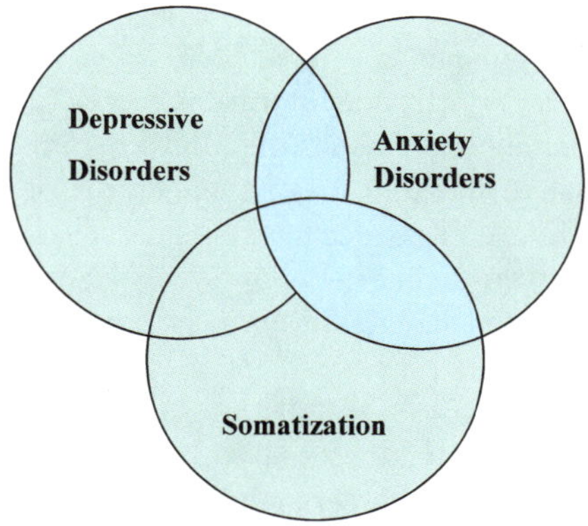

Fig. 11.1 Overlapping of somatization, anxiety and depression

Dissociative Disorders (ICD-10: F 44)

Dissociation means literally 'splitting of the consciousness'. Examples are feelings of alienation, like depersonalization and derealization, loss of memory and escapism, semiconsciousness and non-epileptic convulsions.

These phenomena occur frequently in connection with severe emotional traumata, especially after experiences of violence and sexual abuse. No verbal working out of the event is possible. The traumatic experience is split off and finds expression as fear, states of vegetative tension and in the symptoms described under 'posttraumatic stress disorders'.

Differential Diagnosis

Somatoform symptoms may also be part of an anxiety disorder or depression. Feelings of anxiety or depressive symptoms are not experienced consciously, but are expressed at the physical level. We also speak here of *affect equivalent*. See Fig. 11.1 for the overlapping of somatization, anxiety and depression.

Outlook on DSM-V and ICD-11

The concept of 'medically unexplained systems' fosters the dualism of mind and body. The patient's symptoms are seen either as organic ('medically explained') or 'medically unexplained' which may be taken to imply a psychosocial cause. This is still enshrined in the classification of diseases (ICD, DSM) despite the fact that we know that illness is determined by a mixture of biological, psychological and social factors. To overcome this issue of dualism, there is a need to describe relevant factors on all three dimensions (biological, psychological and social) contributing to the distress and suffering of patients with often multiple somatic symptoms.

The next editions of the diagnostic classification systems DSM-V and ICD-11 are in preparation. Intense discussions are currently being held about the future of the category of 'somatoform disorders'. Critics of the current classification point out that, among other issues, the division into organ-medical and psychological conditions is questionable, the current description of the definition is not culturally sensitive, a number of disorders within the category of somatoform disorders are unreliable, and that the diagnostic criteria of somatization disorder are too narrow.

A result of this criticism is a push for a positive definition of somatoform disorders, including illness perception and illness attribution, illness behaviour, health-related anxiety, emotional distress, disability, quality of life, doctor–patient interaction and health care utilisation. The current proposals by the DSM-V working group suggest that these disorders might be subsumed in the future under the diagnostic label of 'Complex Somatic Symptom Disorders' (CSSD). The following preliminary criteria have been specified for CSSD:

To meet criteria for CSSD, criteria A, B and C must be met:

1. *Somatic symptoms*: One or more somatic symptoms that are distressing and/or result in significant disruption in daily life.
2. *Excessive thoughts, feelings and behaviours related to these somatic symptoms or associated health concerns*: At least two of the following are required to meet this criterion:
   a. High level of health-related anxiety.
   b. Disproportionate and persistent concerns about the medical seriousness of one's symptoms.
   c. Excessive time and energy devoted to these symptoms or health concerns.
3. *Chronicity*: Although any one symptom may not be continuously present, the state of being symptomatic is chronic (at least 6 months).

Frequency and Course

The 12-month prevalence of somatoform disorders in the European adult population is 6.3 % (Wittchen et al. 2011). After anxiety and affective disorders, they are ranked third in terms of frequency of occurrence. Somatoform disorder is diagnosed much more frequently in women than in men.

An American study (Kroenke and Mangelsdorff 1989) examined the proportion of physical diseases for the ten most frequent complaints over a 3-year period. An organic cause was identified in only 16 % of 1,000 patients. Functional somatic symptoms/somatization was probable in a large number of the remaining patients (Fig. 11.2).

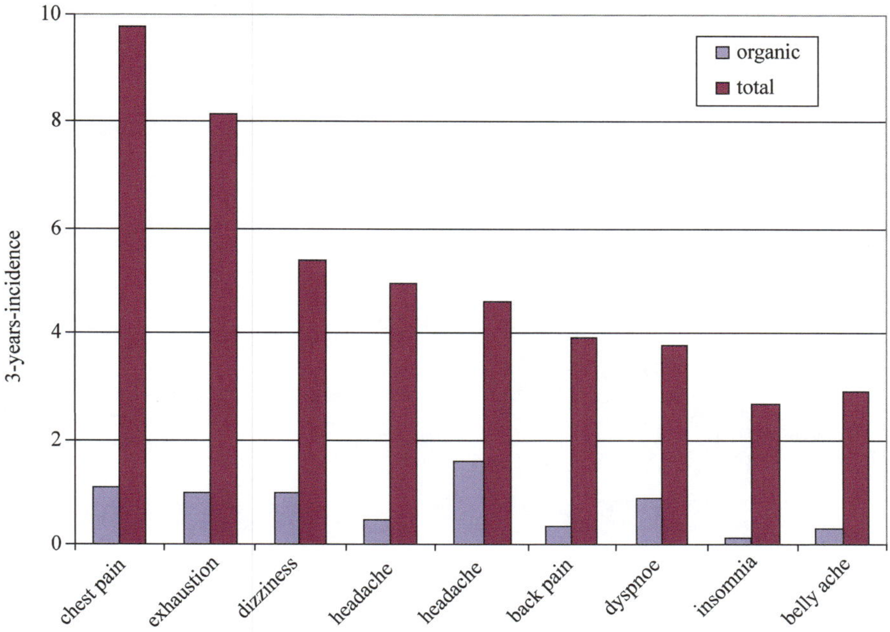

Fig. 11.2 Physical complaints in a 3-year-course

Onset

Every person reacts to emotional stress with physical symptoms, such as sweating, insomnia, palpitations, diarrhoea etc. MUS-patients either do not perceive the emotional stress, or there is inhibition in expressing emotions. The attention is focused instead on the accompanying physical symptoms, which undergo negative assessment and potentiation and are no longer associated with the eliciting feelings. Complaining of the physical pain replaces the expression of unpleasant feelings.

In a *vicious circle,* the physical symptoms increase the fear, which in turn results in greater physical symptoms (Fig. 11.3).

The following *psychosocial factors* promote somatization:

- Traumatization in childhood
- Negative bonding experience
- Model learning from parental models, who experience similar complaints
- Tendency to emotional and physical overtaxing
- Low self-esteem, easily insulted and hurt
- Strengthening of the role of illness with increased attention and support of the environment
- Relief from social or family demands and responsibilities as a result of the complaints

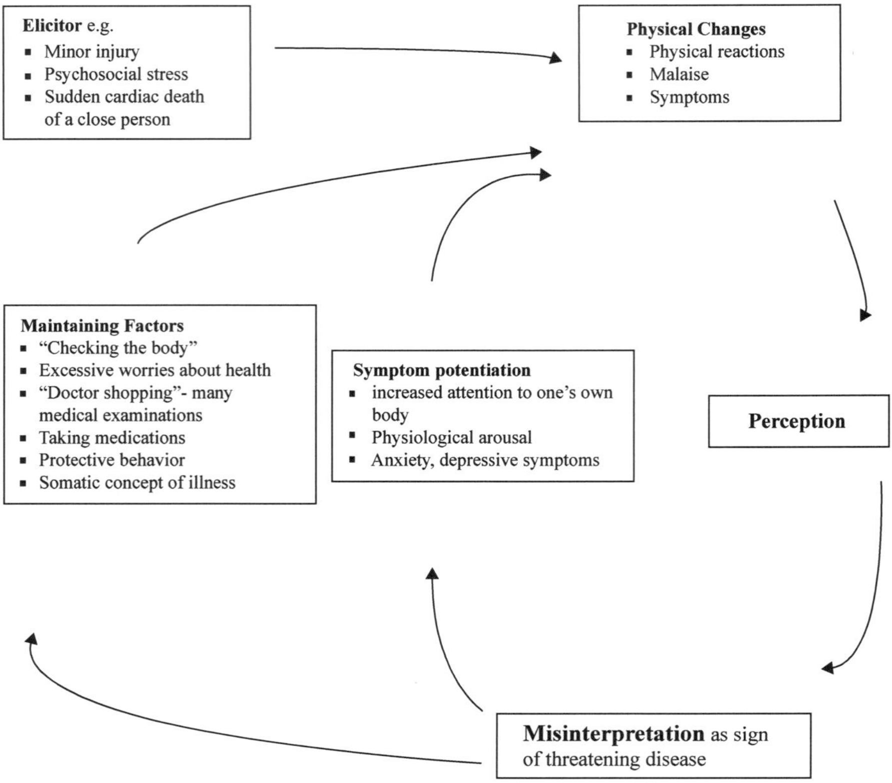

Fig. 11.3 Vicious circle

Practice

Recognition

Signs of somatoform disorders may be:

- The symptoms do not follow anatomic or physiological patterns
- The report of the symptoms is diffuse
- Complaints are accepted without emotion on the one hand, described in dramatic images and inadequate effects on the other
- The patient appears lamenting, demanding clinging
- There are other complaints which cannot be adequately explained organically
- Frequent change of doctor (doctor shopping)
- Current stress, such as at work, or in the family.

Practical Tip: 'Pain History'

- What relieves the pain?
- What aggravates the pain?
- What does a typical day with pain look like?
- Is there a change in pain level during the day?
- When did the pain first occur?
- What kind of experiences with respect to pain are there in the family and personal history?

Basic Therapeutic Attitude

The objective of treatment in psychosomatic primary care is to establish an empathic and trusting doctor–patient relationship, in which the patient feels that he is being taken seriously in his complaints and his view of the illness. After an organic disease has been ruled out, other explanation models can then be discussed and, if necessary, the patient motivated to accept further psychotherapeutic treatment. Treatment goal is relief of complaints, not cure. Regular appointments, e.g. every 14 days, is recommended.

The following belong to a *basic therapeutic attitude:*

- Take the physical complaints seriously
- Understand the patient's helplessness, disappointment and anger
- Even if the doctor does not believe there is an organic cause of disease, the patient should at least undergo brief physical examination
- No precipitous coupling of reported or presumed emotional stress with the physical complaints
- Patience, calmness and knowledge of the limitations of therapeutic possibilities

Basic Interventions

The 3-Stage Model

For treatment in primary care, the *3-stage model* has proven helpful.

Stage 1: Feeling Understood

- Take a full history of the symptoms
- Explore emotional problems
- Explore social and family factors
- Explore symptom beliefs
- Past similar problems and treatment
- Brief, focused physical examination

Following a detailed description of all physical ailments, the doctor elicits the disease and treatment expectations of the patient.

Case Study (continued)
Doctor: What do you think is causing your abdominal pain?
Patient: I know it sounds silly, but my mother had uterine cancer and it started with such abdominal pain. I often think that no one has recognized my cancer yet.
Doctor: Do you worry a lot about it?
Patient: Yes.Doctor: If you agree, I'll examine you physically now.
(continued)

Short, targeted physical examinations, coupled with empathy for the physical symptoms convey to the patient a serious attitude towards his/her physical experience.

The diagnosis should be done as a parallel or simultaneous diagnosis of somatic and psychosocial factors. Even during their first visit, patients should be asked about their mental wellbeing.

Careful physical examination should be repeated at regular intervals, especially with persistent somatoform complaints. In this way, changes in symptoms can be detected in time, it will give the patient a feeling of security and of being taken seriously, and ideally complex instrumental tests are avoided. In case of emerging symptoms, somatic as well as psychosocial diagnosis should be adjusted or extended.

Stage 2: Establish the Agenda Through Negotiation

Objectives of the second treatment step:

- Acknowledge distress or symptoms
- What does the patient want?
- Feedback the results of the examinations

Case Study (continued)
Doctor: The laboratory tests, ultrasound and computer tomography have not shown evidence of an organic disease. I would like to examine your abdomen.... Your abdomen is sensitive in the middle area, but I don't find anything else remarkable. But I can imagine that you suffer a lot from your complaints.
(continued)

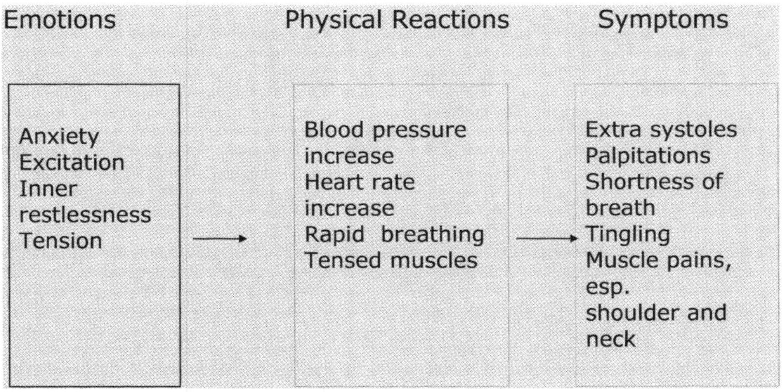

Fig. 11.4 The relationship between anxiety, physiological reaction and somatic symptoms

Stage 3: Making the Link

Objectives of this third treatment step:

- Reframe the complaints: link symptoms with stress or lifestyle
  - Three-level explanation for anxiety (Fig. 11.4)
- Agreement
  - Acknowledge bodily distress
  - Treatment of depression, anxiety
  - Self-management strategies
  - Watchful waiting
  - Psychotherapy

Development of an *alternative model of disease* by explaining psychophysiological relationships, such as between fear and physical symptoms. The following phrases can be used here:

'In frightened people, the body excretes more adrenalin. That's why their hearts beat faster in situations of fear'.

'If people are worried, or are depressed, the intestines can contract and that causes abdominal pain'.

Everyday body-related expressions are especially helpful, such as 'when the heart skips a beat, makes you sick to your stomach, gets under one's skin'.

In this phase, we also recommend the use of a symptom diary (Table 11.3) in which the perception of complaints and their misassessment, such as the fear of having a serious illness, are captured. These cognitive and emotional processing mechanisms can be addressed and discussed during doctor visits, i.e. be placed in new contexts.

Practical Tip: 'Symptom Diary'
'There are a lot of different causes of stomach ache. You see what has already been examined. We'll find the problem together. I would like to get a complete picture again of the complaints you have. Please keep a pain diary until your next appointment'.

Table 11.3 Symptom diary for a better understanding of pain

Day/time	Symptoms/extent of the complaints	Situation, other people, activity, demands	Thoughts in that situation	Feelings and moods in that situation
Monday 10 am	Stomach ache (8)[a] tenesmus (8)	I am giving a sales pitch, another customer wants advice	I must come to an end, otherwise I am losing the other customers	Pressure to perform, fear of failing
Monday 7 pm	Severe abdominal pain (10) tenesmus (9) burning pain with bowel movement (9)	My husband just came home, 2 h late, without explanation and apology	Where has he been? At least he could have called while I'm sitting here alone	Anger, tense atmosphere

[a]Severity 0–10: *0* not at all, *10* very strong and pronounced

The record of thoughts and feelings when abdominal pain and tenesmus appeared are discussed and re-evaluated with the patient.

The links between the appearance of physical symptoms and stressful life situations are explained and the patient is motivated for psychotherapeutic treatment.

Case Study (continued)

Doctor: You mentioned last time that you were having problems at work?

Patient: Yes, some jobs are to be made redundant, and I'm really worried. Sometimes I even cry.

Doctor: I see you're tense and sad at the moment. Physical tension can cause muscle cramps and cause such pain as you are now having.

Patient: You think that's related to my abdominal pain?

Doctor: I think your worries may be affecting your stomach.

Patient: You believe that the muscles in my abdomen are cramping and causing my stomach ache? But my being sad, does that cause pain, too?

Doctor: Yes, of course. Can you relax, for example when you are in bed?

Patient: Oh, no.

Doctor: I think that's a result of the worries you have.Patient: Hmh—could be. But what can I do about it?

Doctor: How do you feel when you talk about it?

Patient: It does me good to show you what I'm feeling and know you'll understand. I try to be strong, but I really have no idea what's going to happen next.

Doctor: I think psychotherapeutic interviews could help you to deal better with your anxieties and worries about your job and help to you relax.

Patient: What do 'psychotherapeutic interviews' mean, exactly?

The occurring stressful emotions are linked to the physical discomfort. Encouragement to verbalize feelings, to express criticism and to assert of one's own position has a relieving and symptom-reducing effect.

Other Treatment Measures

Physical or athletic activation, e.g. aerobic endurance training, active form of physical therapy should be well prepared and accompanied by sustained motivation. The intensity should to be gradually increased, alternating with rest periods.

Drugs, e.g. for the regulation of cardiac dysfunction, symptomatic drug therapy for irritable bowel syndrome and for pain relief should be used only after a critical risk-benefit assessment and only for a limited time.

Psychopharmaceutical Treatment

In more severe, pain-dominant somatoform disorders with and without accompanying depressive symptoms, antidepressants of different classes are moderately effective. For non-pain dominant somatoform complaints additional temporary antidepressants should be given, only in clinically relevant mental comorbidity of anxiety or depression.

Pitfalls

The doctor believes he has recognized the psychosomatic relationships and would like to share his/her knowledge with the patient. However, the patient does not accept the interpretation of the doctor. On the contrary, because of the interpretation of the physician, the patient closes himself/herself even more and increases the presentation of physical complaints. For the treatment, it is important to recognize that one's own understanding is not relevant. The decisive factor is the willingness of the patient to be open to alternative explanations.

The doctor wants to proceed too quickly with the motivation for psychotherapy. The treatment of medical complaints without sufficient medical finding is a very gentle process and requires a lot of sensitivity.

Cooperation

The referral to an outpatient or inpatient psychotherapeutic treatment takes best place as part of a stepped-care model (Table 11.4).

Table 11.4 The stepped-care model in primary and secondary care. (Adapted from Henningsen et al. 2007)

The stepped-care model in primary and secondary care
Step 1
Reassurance with positive explanation of somatoform symptoms
Symptomatic measures like pain relief
Advise graded activation or exercise rather than rest
Advise on dysfunctional attributions and illness behaviour and encourage reframing of symptoms within biopsychosocial framework
If appropriate: appointments at regular intervals rather than patient-initiated
Step 2 (If Step 1 proves to be insufficient)
Prepare referral to psychotherapist or mental-health specialist with reappointment
Consider antidepressant treatment
Ensure that traumatic stressors and maintaining context factors, such as litigation, are assessed
Continue with appointments at regular intervals rather than patient initiated
Liaise with psychotherapist or mental-health specialist on further treatment planning and difficulties

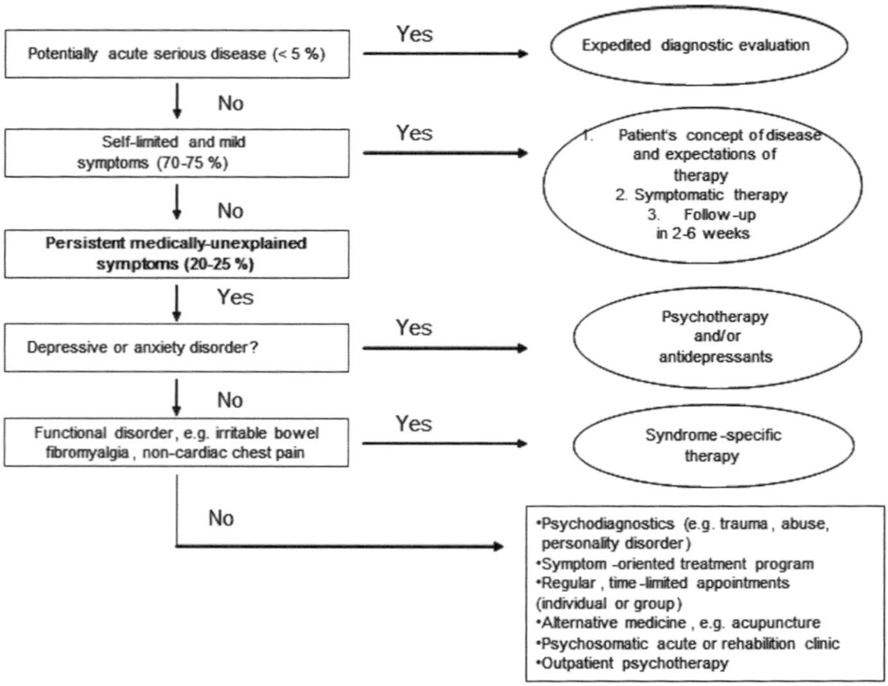

Fig. 11.5 Algorithm of the management of patients with somatic complaints

For deciding which treatment step is appropriate for a patient with unexplained physical symptoms, the algorithm shown in Fig. 11.5 may be used to assist (Kroenke 2003).

Cognitive-behavioural treatment methods are effective in terms of improving the physical comfort, the quality of life and in reducing health care costs. In chronic fatigue syndrome, fibromyalgia and in not organically related heart problems improvements were found on the symptom level. A *psychodynamic treatment approach* has been shown to be effective in patients with functional upper and lower abdominal complaints (irritable bowel syndrome).

Cultural Aspects

Nonspecific, functional and somatoform symptoms occur in all cultures, but differ with respect to the complaint type, the explanatory models, the attribution of importance and expression. In addition, there are 'culture specific syndromes', which exist only within a defined culture. Ethnic minorities and refugees, due to increased psychosocial stress due to emigration, including communication problems, report probably more often about nonspecific functional and somatoform symptoms.

The somatic presentation is part of patient's illness behaviour. It does not necessarily mean that the patient is unable to present emotional problems or does not know how to make psychological complaints. It simply indicates that the patient presents somatic symptoms from numerous reasons, including that he is following a culturally moulded pattern of problem presentation as pointed out by Kirmayer and Young (1998). The presentation of somatic symptoms has multiple indications: It can be seen as an index of a disorder, an indication of a psychopathology, a symbolic condensation of intrapsychic conflicts, a culturally coded expression of distress, a medium for expressing social discontent, and a mechanism through which patients attempt to reposition themselves within their local worlds. That means the nature of somatic presentation needs to be understood and grasped dynamically rather than merely given the label of somatization for somatoform disorders.

The concept and category of 'somatoform disorders' is a product of the contemporary professional orientation, that dichotomatizes the body and mind and categorizes disorders simply by the nature of symptomatic manifestation.

There are no systematic cross-cultural differences in the overall incidence of somatoform symptoms (Gureje et al. 1997; Kirmayer and Young 1998). The irritable bowel syndrome seems to be more common in Western cultures than in non-Western (Chang et al. 2006), as well as multiple chemical sensitivity or the sensitivity to amalgam (Hausteiner et al. 2005).

In Latin American countries and also in other countries, the concept regarding the causes of different diseases varies considerable between traditional medicine and formal medicine. Although there is a direct and mutual influence among both systems in terms of the diagnosis and treatment processes of any disease, popular treatments are not limited to professionally defined diseases but deal to a large extend with psychosocial and emotional conditions. What health professionals describe as specific diseases are not necessarily aligned with diseases defined by the popular knowledge. The decision of the patient of seeing a doctor or a healer depends on factors including perception of the cause of the disease, severity of the disease and accessibility to health services.

Somatic Symptoms as Cultural Idioms of Distress (Iran)

The idiom of 'heart distress' among Iranians can be understood as a culturally prescribed way of talking about a host of personal and social concerns primarily related to loss and grief (Laurence and Young 1998). Many Iranian people complain of tensions, distress and worries by words related to 'heart'. The word 'del' is used by people pointing to both heart and abdomen. Both parts of the body are the origin of many discomforts. 'Del dard' refers to abdominal pain and discomfort, though 'dard e del' means telling some secrets or ventilation due to tensions or sad events. So, many psychosomatic complaints are related to 'del'. Although the patient's narrative of his or her illness may include a significant subtext, it links his or her physical distress to social predicaments, moral sentiments and otherwise unexpressed emotions. Throughout the Middle-East, reference to the heart is commonly understood not just as potential signs of illness but as natural metaphors for a range of emotions.

Somatic complaints are the most common and important causes of visits in different clinics (Ahmadzadeh and Masodzadeh 1997). Variety and number of somatic complaints of patients who visited psychiatric clinics are more than of patients who are referred to medical and dermatologic clinics. In several studies, the main complaints in depressive patients were somatic complaints. The most common complaints in psychiatric clinics are headaches, muscular and joint pains, generalized fatigue, palpitation and GI complaints. Somatic presentation is the most common presentation of depressive disorders in the Iranian patient population. Somatic presentations are more common in depressed women, in the geriatric population and in low-socioeconomic groups. Fear of stigmatization and acceptance of somatic complaints instead of emotional expression and verbalization of affective suffering are the principle cause of this phenomenon.

Certainly, most of the psychiatric patients who visited a psychiatrist for the first time, had visited general practitioners and other specialists due to somatic complaints which causes unnecessary workups and spending resources, and finally a delay in diagnosis and mismanagement in this group.

Neurasthenia (China)

The term neurasthenia was introduced in the USA by New York neurologist George M. Beard in 1869 (Beard 1869). It was very popular at the time and included about 30 symptoms. The diagnostic concept spread around the world, and it was referred to as shenjing shuairuo in China and shinkei shuijaku in Japan. Shenjing shuairuo includes somatic, cognitive and emotional symptoms. Patients whose clinical picture included sleep disorders, dizziness, headaches, concentration disorders, rapid exhaustion and many other similar symptoms very often received this diagnosis (Kleinman 1982; Yan 1991). Despite its origin in Western psychiatry, shenjing shuairuo has become a popular concept in Chinese folk medicine.

Symptoms such as weakness and exhaustion are important in traditional Chinese medicine, and they are related to a lack of 'qi' or hypofunctioning of 'kidney', imbalance between 'yin and yang', hyperfunctioning of 'liver', or imbalance between the function of 'kidney' and 'heart'. Its origin was regarded as organic, but the treatment consists of psychological and social therapies such as traditional Chinese medicinal herbs, acupuncture, qi gong and shadow-boxing. In addition, drug therapy, physical therapy and group psychotherapy were used after a philosophical and medical consideration of patients. The concept of shenjing shuairuo additionally has the advantage not to be stigmatising.

In 2001, the concept of somatoform disorders was introduced into the Chinese Classification of Mental Disorders (CCMD-III). At the same time, hierarchical rules were established permitting the diagnosis of shenjing shuairuo only after exclusion of depressive disorders and anxiety disorders. Neurasthenia received code 43.5 in the CCMD-III and therefore ranked behind other forms of somatoform disorders. As a result, shenjing shuairuo is now rarely diagnosed by Chinese psychiatrists. However, in neurological and general hospitals outside the major urban centres, the diagnosis is still used.

Dissociative Disorder and Pain Disorder in Vietnam

Symptoms of dissociative disorder are functional paralysis and loss of voice. Recently, trance and possession disorder has been seen in Vietnam. In this state, the dead person invades patients and helps their alive relatives to find out the place of his/her grave.

Somatized pain disorder is often seen. Pain usually occurs in chest, head, joint etc. Stomach, intestinal and muscular disturbances are detected as their symptoms. The relation between pain and other somatic disorders as cardiologic disorders, endocrinologic disorders etc., is unexplained. Patients with these disorders often go to somatic departments first. They usually go to see psychiatrist later. According to some studies, somatized disorder was recognized after 2–2.5 years of onset.

Psychopharmacology is of common use in psychiatry. Using psychotherapy among these patients is still limited because lacking of experts and clinical psychologists in Vietnam.

Body Dismorphic Disorder (Latin America)

In tropical countries, such as the Latin American continent, where more exposure of the body happens, research evidenced a high prevalence of Body Dismophic Disorder (dismorphia), which concerns with body shape and skin perfection. It ranges from 1 to 2 % in the general population and it gets as high as 16 % in dermatological and cosmetic surgery patients. The majority of the patients experience some degree of impairment in social or occupational functioning, and obsessive thoughts may lead to repetitive behaviours and to attempted suicide in the more severe cases. Research findings show that most individuals have poor insight and cannot acknowledge that what they indeed need is psychiatric treatment because their physical problem is indeed minimal or inexistent. The most frequent dermatological concerns are dyschromias, acne, the shape of the body and ageing. Research has also evidenced that a reasonable number of patients had already performed clinical or surgical treatments with poor results. Moreover, some comorbidities were encountered such as: major depressive disorders and obsessive compulsive disorders.

Other examples of culture-specific syndromes that can broadly be considered somatoform disorders include:

Brain-fag (Nigeria)

'Brain-fag', first described in 1960 in southern Nigeria (Prince 1960): cognitive impairments, visual and other sensory disturbances and various physical complaints, mainly burning pain in the head and neck area. Brain fag is subjectively attributed to mental stress (Tseng 2006).

Dhat (India, Nepal, Pakistan, Bangladesh and Sri Lanka)

Various body symptoms such as fatigue, weakness, loss of appetite, sexual dysfunction, caused apparently by nocturnal loss of semen in the urine (Tseng 2006). (see also chapter anxiety disorder).

Arctic Hysteria (Greenland)

'Pibloktoq' or 'Arctic Hysteria', first described in 1913 in Northwest Greenland: Sudden consciousness disorders up to the loss of consciousness associated with behavioural problems such as tearing clothes off the body, swearing, tossing objects, mostly occurring in women in the Arctic winter, most likely under extreme physical and psychological stress, but was also attributed to hyperglycaemia or hypervitaminosis A (Tseng 2006).

Pain Syndrome (East Africa)

'Hapa na Hap' Syndrome means pains here and here. A description of somatisation symptoms such as headaches, tiredness, constipation, or other unspecific symptoms, commonly by health workers in Kenya (Jenkins et al. 2010).

References

Ahmadzadeh GH, Masodzadeh A. The major complaints in depression. J Isfahan Med Sch. 1997;46:61–6.

Beard G. Neurasthenia or nervous exhaustion. Boston Med Surg J. 1869;3:217–20.

Chang L, Toner BB, Fukudo S, Guthrie E, Locke GR, Norton, NJ, et al. Gender, age society, culture, and the patient's perspective in the functional gastrointestinal disorders. Gastroenterology. 2006;130(5):1435–46.

Gureje O, Simon GE, Ustun TB, Goldberg DP. Somatization in cross-cultural perspective: a World Health Organization study in primary care. Am J Psychiatry. 1997;154(7):989–95.

Hausteiner C, Bormschein S, Hansen J, Zilker T, Förstl H. Self-reported chemical sensitivity in Germany: a population-based survey. Int J Hyg Environ Health. 2005;208(4):271–8.

Henningsen P, Zipfel S, Herzog W. Management of functional somatic syndromes. Lancet 2007;369:946–55.

Jenkins R, Kiima D, Okonji M, Njenga F, Kingora J, Lock S. Integration of mental health into primary care and community health working in Kenya: context, rationale, coverage and sustainability. Ment Health Fam Med. 2010;7(1):37–47.

Kirmayer LJ, Young A. Culture and somatization: clinical, epidemiological. and ethnographic perspectives. Psychosom Med. 1998;60(4):420–30.

Kleinman AM. Neurasthenia and depression: a study of somatization and culture in China. Cult Med Psychiatry. 1982;6:1170–90.

Kroenke K, Mangelsdorff AD. Common symptoms in ambulatory care: incidence, evaluation, therapy, and outcome. Am J Med. 1989;86(3):262–6.

Kroenke K. Patients presenting with somatic complaints: epidemiology, psychiatric comorbidity and management. Int J Methods Psychiatr Res. 2003;12:34–43.

Laurence J, Young A. Culture and somatization: Clinical, Epidemiological and Ethnographic Perseptives. Psychosom Med. 1998;60:420–30.

Prince R. The "brain fag" syndrome in Nigerian students. J Med Sci. 1960;106:559–70.

Tseng WS. From peculiar psychiatric disorders through culture-bound syndromes to culture-related specific syndromes. Transcult Psychiatry. 2006;43(4):554–76.

Wittchen HU, Jacobi F, Rehm J, Gustavsson A, Svensson M, Jönsson B, et al. The size and burden of mental disorders and other disorders of the brain in Europe 2010. Eur Neuropsychopharmacol. 2011;21:655–79.

Yan HQ. Neurasthenia in China. Psychiat Ann. 1991;22:188–9.

Chapter 12
Psycho-Oncology

Kurt Fritzsche, Gertrud Frahm, Sonia Diaz Monsalve, Hamid Afshar Zanjani and Farzad Goli

Case Study A 55-year-old Mr. M. is hospitalized because of intractable cough. The medical history shows that since his 18th year of age Mr. M. has smoked, on average, 20 cigarettes per day, until 5 years ago. He is married (two adult children), an electrician by profession and works as a clerk in a small business.

Chest X-ray and chest CT scan are showing a mass, the bronchoscopic biopsy indicates small cell lung cancer.

The patient comes "to discuss the findings". Spontaneously he says:

K. Fritzsche (✉) · S. D. Monsalve
Department of Psychosomatic Medicine and Psychotherapy,
University Medical Center, Hauptstr. 8, 79104 Freiburg, Germany
e-mail: kurt.fritzsche@uniklinik-freiburg.de

S. D. Monsalve
e-mail: sonia.diaz-monsalve@uniklinik-freiburg.de

G. Frahm
Department of Human Sciences, Federal University of Paraná,
R. Gal. Carneiro, 460, Curitiba, PR 80060-150, Brazil
e-mail: gfrahm@uol.com.br

H. Afshar Zanjani
Department of Psychiatry, Medical Faculty, Isfahan University of Medical Sciences,
Isfahan 81736-44165, Iran
e-mail: afshar@med.mui.ac.ir, shafsharz@gmail.com

Noor Hospital, Isfahan, Iran

F. Goli
Department of bioenergy economy, Energy Medicine University, California, USA
e-mail: Dr.fgoli@yahoo.com

Danesh-e Tandorosti Institute, Isfahan, Iran
e-mail: info@iranianhealth.com

K. Fritzsche et al. (eds.), *Psychosomatic Medicine,* DOI 10.1007/978-1-4614-1022-5_12,

> "These many examinations have made me increasingly scared. Four months ago, when I spat blood, I knew: Now you have cancer!"
> (continued)

Definition

Cancer is a disease which in 50 % of cases is fatal and whose treatment is highly stressful both physically and mentally. Generally, cancer triggers anxiety and helplessness, the disease is often equated with death and dying. The diagnosis is an intrusion into the structure of life of the individual which may affect the entire family.

Psycho-oncology deals with the influence of emotional and social factors on the onset of disease, its course and how patients cope with it, and examines the effectiveness of psychotherapeutic treatments in improving the patient's emotional well-being and quality of life.

Relevance

Psychosocial support is reasonable and necessary if the extent of stress exceeds the coping ability of patients and families and affects the mental state and social relationships. Depending on the disease and treatment stage, this is the case in 30–50 % of all patients with a diagnosis of cancer. These patients exhibit—at least immediately after the diagnosis—clinically significant symptoms of a mental disorder, usually in the form of anxiety and depressive symptoms with rumination and sleep disorders and/or with physical limitations during radiotherapy and chemotherapy such as pain, nausea and fatigue.

Theory

Symptoms

The mental problems in cancer are not fundamentally different from those in other serious physical illnesses. For attending doctors, nurses and relatives, it is important to realize that most patients are not primarily mentally ill, rather their mental problems concern mainly emotional reactions, mostly anxiety, depression, resentment and anger at the diagnosis of cancer. The symptoms accumulate during the first weeks after diagnosis and become less thereafter. In a small number of patients they may last for another year or two.

Table 12.1 shows typical emotional reactions and challenges in the course of cancer that the concerned persons have to deal with.

Table 12.1 Mental reactions occurring in the course of cancer and tasks ahead

Illness phase	Mental reaction	Tasks to be managed by the patient
Diagnosis	Shock, fear	Accepting the diagnosis, coping with intense emotions
	Disbelief, despair, depression	Making a decision regarding treatment
	Anger	Notifying the social environment
Primary treatment phase	Anxiety, depression, loss of control and autonomy	Accepting illness and treatment
	Loss of physical integrity	Coping with treatment side effects
	Loneliness, loss of intimacy and sexual contacts	Establishment of viable relationships with the treatment team
		Regaining mental and physical self-esteem
Remission	Relief, gratitude	Return to everyday life, living with uncertainty
	Fear of recurrence and metastases, increased awareness of the body	Development of new perspectives on life, return to work
Recurrence	Shock, anxiety, depression	Accepting uncertainty of the future
	Denial	Accepting the progression of the disease and the likelihood of death
	Loss of hope and trust	Adaptation of the perspective of life to the new situation
	Increased vulnerability	
	Search for meaning, feelings of guilt	
Terminal stage	Fear of death, depression, demoralization	Dealing with death and dying, mourning the loss
	Denial	Accepting one's own death
	Loss of control	Accepting the physical decline and the prognosis
	Fear of loneliness	Arrangement of family affairs and legal matters and, parting from family and friends
	Increasing dependence on doctors and nursing staff	Looking back at one's own life, dealing with spiritual issues
	Retreat	
	Anger and resentment	

Diagnostic Categories

In the spectrum of mental disorders, the following diagnostic categories are mostly relevant in the context of cancer.

Acute Stress Disorder (ICD-10: F43.0)

A transient disorder, in a person who is apparently not mentally disturbed, develops in response to exceptional physical or mental stress, and which generally subsides within hours or days. The symptoms show a mixed and changing picture, starting with a kind of "stunning", with a degree of narrowing of consciousness and limited attention, an inability to process stimuli and disorientation. This state may be followed by a further retreat from the social environment, or a state of restlessness and overactivity. Frequently, vegetative signs of panic anxiety such as tachycardia, sweating and blushing occur.

Adjustment Disorder (ICD-10: F43.2)

The symptoms include depressed mood, anxiety or worry. Particularly, in adolescents, social conduct disorders may be an additional symptom. A difference is made between short depressive and anxiety reactions, which do not last longer than 1 month, and longer reactions, which do not last longer than 2 years.

Problem "Fatigue"

Fatigue is expressed as great tiredness and exhaustion, reduced performance capacity and muscular weakness. It affects especially patients after radiation or chemotherapy. Ca. 30–40 % of patients suffer from chronic fatigue even after the treatment phase has been completed. Even when there is an overlap with depressive symptoms, fatigue is considered a syndrome in its own right. The basis is probably a complex interaction between the tumour disease, chemo- and radiotherapy, tumour anaemia, other secondary diseases, immunological processes and emotional coping processes.

Frequency

Especially in the first weeks after learning the diagnosis or in case of recurrence, 30–50 % of patients show symptoms of emotional distress. Usually this is an acute stress reaction with anxiety and depressive symptoms (see diagnostic categories). Psychiatric disorders in the strict sense are rare.

Onset and Course

Risk factors for mental decompensation in diagnosis or in case of recurrence include previous and current mental problems (especially depression, alcoholism, earlier suicide attempts), lack of social integration and support, current experience of separation and/or death, marriage and family problems, financial and professional problems, negative experiences of illness, uncontrollable pain, poor prognosis, an advanced tumour and physical and emotional exhaustion.

The course of mental well-being during cancer disease depends on the coping mechanisms that are available to a patient. The following coping forms have been found to be favourable:

- An active confrontation with the disease (so-called fighting spirit)
- Search for meaning and spirituality
- Good interpersonal relationships and social support
- Trust in the doctors

Unfavourable coping forms are:

- Passive acceptance, resignation
- Social withdrawal and isolation
- Helplessness and hopelessness

Studies have shown that the availability of a wide range of disease-coping strategies and the targeted use, depending on the situation, enables a better adaptation to the disease process than the prevalence of only one strategy.

Practice

Recognition

The indication for psychosocial care of cancer patients results from the bio-psychosocial history.

Indications for Psychosomatic Basic Care

- Anxiety and depressive reactions after receiving the diagnosis, or as part of therapy
- Suicidality
- Psycho-vegetative reactions such as nausea, weakness and fatigue, sleep and concentration problems (Fatigue syndrome)
- Mental impairments and conflicts in the partnership, such as after surgery
- Avoiding the public by face and larynx-operated patients, or after breast cancer
- Changing roles in the family
- Physically unexplained pain syndromes persisting for a long time despite symptomatic measures
- Posttraumatic stress disorder, for example, after surgery with lots of complications

Basic Therapeutic Attitude

There is a very crucial balance between hope and acceptance. Hope, as positive anticipation, could promote the psychoneuroimmunologic system but without acceptance it may lead to an anxious attitude and aversive strategy and finally fade the hope of course in a very tragic way.

Acceptance of the reality of handicaps and death is a humanistic and existential point in cancer condition but without hope it can lead us to a passive and fatalistic attitude.

The doctor accepts the patient, even if he/she does not want to accept the knowledge of his disease. The doctor is not misled about the potentially powerful inner emotional involvement of the patient by the patient's trivializing, indifference and silence. Fear, despair, gloom, withdrawal, anger and rage are considered adequate responses to the diagnosis. The aim is for the patient to be able to cope better with the disease. The patient regains control of his/her thoughts, his/her feelings and his/her behaviour and develops overall an active, problem-oriented attitude.

Basic Interventions

Information and Consultation (Psycho-education)

The first stage includes information and consultation of patients and their families about the disease and the resulting treatment measures with the aim of reducing helplessness and uncertainty due to lack of knowledge. Patients are encouraged to ask questions, to express fantasies of cancer development (subjective theory of disease) and the progression of the disease, and to talk about upsetting thoughts and feelings. This first stage should be offered to all patients after cancer diagnosis either as individual consultation or as part of a group counselling program. It requires basic knowledge of psycho-oncology and psychosomatic primary care.

Specific Measures for Pain, Fatigue, Nausea and Vomiting

For this, there are a wide range of intervention options: Progressive muscle relaxation, autogenic training, hypnosis, deep breathing, meditation, biofeedback, passive relaxation and fantasy trips (so-called guided imagination or visualization). Another common problem with chemotherapy is the anticipatory vomiting and nausea. These side effects follow the rules of classical conditioning and can be influenced by a desensitization treatment. The main objective of these symptom-oriented methods is the development of positive ideas and pleasant body sensations. The techniques used also strengthen mental coping skills and increase self-control. The effectiveness of a combination of progressive muscle relaxation and imaginative techniques could be demonstrated in the reduction of pain in mucositis, a very common and painful complication of chemotherapeutic treatment (Syrjala et al. 1992).

Objectives of a Psychosomatic Co-Treatment

- Giving information to reduce anxiety, despair and depression in patients and relatives

- Crisis intervention suicidality
- Improved compliance with respect to the medical treatment
- Activation of one's own resources for coping with disease
- Learning of behavioural techniques and approaches to better manage and accept the disease
- Learning of relaxation techniques to reduce insomnia, pain, nausea and other physical symptoms
- Breaking the taboo of dying

Breaking Bad News

More than 90 % of all cancer patients in Western countries want to be informed about the disease and possible treatments. An important component of the explanation discussion is the emotional support in dealing with the information. This difficult task requires adequate preparation of the attending doctor.

Setting and Preparation

The announcement of bad news is always made in person whenever possible, in a suitable enclosed space, and in an atmosphere of trust. Before the start of the conversation it is clarified, whether the patient is ready to receive the news. The doctor makes sure that the test results are complete, he/she has understood them and he/she knows how to proceed in the conversation. The doctor also finds out beforehand whether the presence of family is desirable.

Checklist

- Do you have all the test results on hand?
- Has a plan been set up for treatment, for control examinations or further diagnostic steps?
- What do I want to tell the patient concretely?
- Where should I start?

Course of Conversation

- *Patient's perception and information need*

Joining ("How have you been since the last examination? How are you today?") *objective* of the upcoming conversation ("I want to discuss the results of the examination with you") and setting the *timetable* ("We have about half an hour.").

Patient's subjective *status of information,* his *wish for information* and what he thinks about *treatment* ("What do you know about your disease? Do you want as much information as possible or are you a person who would rather not know everything? Have you thought about what will happen next?")

- *Provide knowledge*

Information About the Disease ("I'm sorry but I am afraid I have some bad news. Based on the examination we suspect that you may suffer from cancer.").

Time for Questions from the Patient

- *Responding to emotions with empathy*

Emotional Involvement Conversation techniques that reflect open or perceived feelings are helpful here ("This makes you very depressed and confused. I have the impression that you are angry because you have not been told you earlier that it could be cancer.") Talk about *treatment options* if desired by the patient ("Let me tell you about the treatment possibilities. . .").

- *Summary* of the conversation
- *Support* for the following hours and the way home

Support Informing Family

Set *specific date* to discuss specific questions and treatment plan ("If you have no further questions, we can stop here. I can well imagine that a lot will occur to you later. If you want, we can meet again this evening (tomorrow morning) and talk some more about it.").

- Adapt your information to the patients' speech
- Explain complex information in pictures and make reference to the patient's everyday experience
- Do not make the word cancer a taboo, but watch the patient's reaction and adapt your language to his reaction
- Refer to the emotional reactions of the patient and the family members, do not switch immediately to "facts" when emotionally difficult situations arise
- Silence and pauses with concurrent physical and mental presence is more effective than talking excessively
- Always leave room for hope but do not raise false hope
- Assure reliable, competent and best-possible treatment
- Check repeatedly whether the patient has understood the information
- Inform the patient that he can contact the nursing staff or the doctor on duty if needed

After the Conversation

After the conversation all people involved in treatment (doctors, nurses, physiotherapists, etc.) should be informed. A conversation with a colleague over the course of the conversation and your own feelings to relieve stress serves your own mental health.

Case Study (Continued) A 55-year-old Mr. M. was diagnosed with small cell lung cancer. The attending doctor asks the patient whether it was okay if his wife would join the conversation and, after the patient's consent, asks the patient together with his wife to the doctor's office to inform them of the findings.

Before the conversation, the doctor thinks about what exactly she wants to tell Mr. M. Ideally, she would like to phrase the findings so that Mr. M. still has hope, i.e. offering the possibility of radio- and chemotherapy, and tell him that there is a chance to control associated symptoms such as pain and shortness of breath. She also realizes that she must explain the findings and the treatment to couple M. in simple terms. In any event she does not want to share a prognosis because she knows on the one hand from her own experience that they rarely come true, and on the other, would like to prevent Mr. and Mrs. M. to lose hope.

In the conversation, the ward doctor tries to communicate the findings in a straightforward manner and to remain objective, yet approachable. She tries to dampen the initial shock, by building confidence in the treatment options. She avoids foreign words and explains to the couple M. particularly the treatment options and their mechanism of action as accurately as possible.

It is difficult for Mr. M. to follow the explanations of the doctor. Sometimes he feels numb. Towards the end of the conversation he finally dares to ask whether he has to die now. At first, the doctor is surprised about the directness of this question. Through empathetic inquiries she learns of the painful death of a co-worker and understands the background of the question. Gently, she addresses the fears of the patient and assures him that everything is done to help him and to avoid unnecessary pain and suffering.

Preparing for Death

> Why don't the doctors understand the importance of just being there?
> Why can't they see that the moment in which they can offer nothing more is the moment in which one needs them most? (Paula in Yalom 1999)

Hope is usually associated with a positive goal and success orientation, e.g. reduced to the formulation "with favourable prognosis". It appears as though failure would rule out hope. Giving hope is an important dimension in creating the doctor–patient relationship. Cancer patients, whose legitimate hope for cure and recovery is disappointed, are not necessarily without hope. The hope of survival fades, other hope, such as a peaceful death, reconciliation with estranged family members, or wishes like seeing the new-born grandchild once more become more important. Many dying people show a recovered equilibrium in this extreme situation, with great calmness, wisdom and humour which amazes the outsider. To develop these capabilities, respectful, empathetic attendance is necessary. The dying person needs the feeling that he is not abandoned.

It must be clear to the doctor, that he will experience an intensive, emotional bonding with the patient who is preparing for death. Earlier experience with dying friends, siblings or parents is reactivated. It is important for the doctor to recognize his own "weak points" and vulnerabilities. Doctors who have experienced traumas and loss in their own lives are best in position to empathize and to recognize their limits. They can best understand what it means to prepare for one's own death.

Pitfalls

- The doctor continues to talk, even if the patient is no longer receptive
- There is too much information per time unit
- He/she ignores the patient's emotional reactions
- The doctor quickly changes to the factual level, because he/she no longer can take the emotionally stressful situation and feels overwhelmed to care for the patient long term.
- The doctor gives in to the pressure of the patient or the family, and prescribes a new chemotherapy cycle, although he/she is not convinced of the indication. In the short term, this calms down the situation, but moves all questions related to further tumour growth and the end of life to a time when the course of the disease has worsened and reached a critical state and little time to sort out all the above questions remains. It is merely an evasion of answering vital questions by physician, patient and relatives.

Cooperation

Psychotherapeutic support is appropriate and necessary when the extent of stress exceeds the patient's coping possibilities with detriment to the emotional wellbeing and social relationships over a longer period. This is the case in ca. 10–20 % of all cancer patients. For these patients, depending on the severity of psychosocial stress and motivation, there is a need for treatment which is graded in intensity and duration. Emotionally stressed partners, children and other persons close to the patient are part of the target group.

Indication

Psychotherapeutic treatment by psychiatrist or psychological psychotherapists is indicated in:

- Suicidal tendency (see Chap. 9 "Depressive Disorders")
- Latent conflicts or personality disorders (ICD-10: F60, F61, F63) which became manifest through the cancer disease
- Emotional disorders existing for a longer period, e.g. depression (ICD-10: F32, F34), anxiety disorder (ICD-10: F40, F41), psychosis (ICD-10: F06, F2), which become worse due to the traumatic effect of learning the diagnosis and which make adaption to the disease situation more difficult
- Posttraumatic stress reactions (ICD-10: F43.1), e.g. after bone marrow transplantation with complications

The efficacy of psychoeducative and psychotherapeutic treatment procedures in the improvement of wellbeing and quality of life is considered proven. It could also be shown that painful states, nausea and vomiting, as side effects of chemotherapy, can be influenced by cognitive-behavioural techniques and imagination procedures. The influence of psychotherapy on the course of the disease and survival time is probably very slight and has not yet been convincingly demonstrated.

In many hospitals, there is a psychiatric and psychosomatic consulting and liaison service which takes over the specialist psychotherapeutic treatment and conducts courses to support doctors and nurses in learning the basic psychosomatic competence.

Cultural Aspects

Patients of different societies react differently to the disease of cancer. American patients mostly held views of adaption and hope. African patients maintained more fatalistic and powerless views. The Latin model associated breast trauma and "bad" behaviours as risk factors for breast cancer. How the major problem and its symptoms are described are subject to the patient's educational level, medical knowledge and culturally patterned modes. Chinese people describe a depressed mood as "I feel my heart is empty", without any cardiac problem. A culturally sensitive physician will try to understand the symbolic meaning behind what is said rather than taking the complaint exactly. Furthermore, patient's relation with the medical team may be different. Japanese patients will try to ask the nurses, with whom they feel more comfortable sharing any problems. In Western societies they expect that a person have an established family physician, but in Asian countries, a patient will shop around for physicians without feeling a commitment to remain with any particular family physician.

There also exists a wide range as to whether the physician should truthfully inform the patient about the diagnosis. The way to deliver bad news is influenced by cultural aspects (Ong et al. 2002). In many Western countries, oncologists usually inform cancer patients about their cancer diagnosis (Grassi et al. 2000); 98 % of patients would like to know their diagnosis, and 87 % of patients would like to receive all available information, both good and bad (Jenkins et al. 2001). The individual need of the patient is highly respected. The ethical principle of autonomy integrates this approach (Beauchamp and Childress 2001).

However, it needs to be pointed out that in the USA and other Western countries it was not common to practice disclosure of "bad news" about terminal illness prior to the 1960s. Currently, disclosure of medical information to patients is necessary because of the physician's concerns about malpractice suits and the legal need to obtain the patient's consent to treatment.

But until today there exist widely different cultural views as to whether the physician should truthfully inform the patient about the diagnosis of a life-threatening disease.

Patient from different ethnic backgrounds react differently to the fatal disease of cancer. Patients from Western countries mostly held views of adaption and hope. Patients from Africa and Asia maintained more fatalistic and powerless views.

Asia

For Asian physicians, disclosing diagnosis and prognosis to patients represents a big challenge, because they are confronted with a family-centred model of decision-making (Back and Huak 2005). Accordingly, it is expected that physicians first talk to family members, who then decide whether the patient should be informed or not. Mostly, it is the task of senior physicians and it is seen as a sign of competence and respect. If a junior or a nurse broke bad news directly to the patients, it would be seen as a reduction of trust and might cause dissatisfaction. However, junior physicians and nurses are expected to give more detailed information to patients afterwards, to be in charge for the patients throughout treatment and for counselling. Most Asian families, however, ask physicians not to reveal the diagnosis and prognosis to patients (Hu et al. 2002). One reason for that might be the fear of families that their family member suffering from cancer would be in despair and might commit suicide (Tse et al. 2003).

This approach places emphasis on keeping patients away from harms and is integrated in the ethical principle of beneficence (Beauchamp and Childress 2001). However, more and more patients in Asia would like to be fully informed and the right of being informed has been regulated by law. This new development represents a dilemma for oncologists. On the one hand they have to respect patients' autonomy and on the other hand they need to consider families' concerns about beneficence (Wang et al. 2004).

Iran

Several studies conducted in Iran demonstrated that cancer is a taboo subject and the word cancer, as well as other indicative terms, were rarely used in daily communication. A climate of nondisclosure predominated because patients were the last to know their diagnosis, they were unaware of their prognosis, and family members and physicians employed strategies to conceal this information. The mutual concern of patients, family members and physicians was the main reason that cancer was not discussed (Zamanzadeh et al. 2011).

Latin America

In most Latin American countries, cancer is highly stigmatized and viewed as a "death sentence", with a culture of silence and fatalism implying that there is no treatment that can change the outcome of death. Given income inequalities and the weak health infrastructure, often the treatment options are limited. Perceptions of cancer (cause and treatment) vary with educational ranks, social levels and access to early detection and treatment services.

A research developed in Cuba with 98 doctors, in situation of serious illnesses communication, has shown that the prevalent doctor–patient relationship mode is an active-passive or a top-down paternalistic approach. This mode has shown preference not to communicate bad news to the patient with avoidance of reporting the truth about the illness. Also, among others, lack of empathy and mutual trust in the communication process was evidenced, as well as lack of exploration on what the patient already knew of the illness and of what the patient wanted to know. This research study revealed that a great number of the doctors surveyed did not have adequate communication skills (Martinez and Trujilo 2009).

References

Back MF, Huak CY. Family centred decision making and non-disclosure of diagnosis in a South East Asian oncology practice. Psychooncology. 2005;14:1052–9.

Beauchamp TL, Childress F. Principles of biomedical ethics. 5th ed. New York: Oxford University Press; 2001.

Grassi L, Giraldi T, Messina EG, Magnani K, Valle E, Cartei G. Physicians' attitudes to and problems with truth-telling to cancer patients. Support Care Cancer. 2000;8:40–5.

Hu WY, Chiu TY, Chuang RB, Chen CY. Solving family-related barriers to truthfulness in cases of terminal cancer in Taiwan. A professional perspective. Cancer Nurs. 2002;25:486–92.

Jenkins V, Fallowfield L, Saul J. Information needs of patients with cancer: results from a large study in UK cancer centres. Br J Cancer. 2001;84:48–51.

Martinez HI, Trujilo MC. Communicating bad news to patients with neurodegenerative diseases: physitians/ skills. Revista Latinoamericana de Bioética. 2009;9:76–85.

Ong KJ. Back MF, Lu JJ, Shakespeare TS, Wynne CJ. Cultural attitudes to cancer management in traditional South-East-Asian patients. Australas Radiol. 2002;46:370–4.

Syrjala KL, Cummings C, Donaldson GW. Hypnosis or cognitive behavioral training for the reduction of pain and nausea during cancer treatment: a controlled clinical trial. Pain. 1992;50:237–8.

Tse CY, Chong A, Fok SY. Breaking bad news: a Chinese perspective. Palliat Med. 2003;17:339–43.

Wang SY, Chen CH, Chen YS, Huang HL. The attitude toward truth telling of cancer in Taiwan. J Psychosom Res. 2004;57:53–8.

Yalom ID. Travels with Paula. In: Yalom ID, editor. Momma and the meaning of life. New York: Basis books; 1999.

Zamanzadeh V, Rahmani A, Valizadeh L, Ferguson C, Hassankhani H, Nikanfar AR, Howard F. The taboo of cancer: the experiences of cancer disclosure by Iranian patients, their family members and physicians. Psychooncology. 2011;21:1002–10.

Chapter 13
Psycho-Cardiology

Kurt Fritzsche, Gertrud Frahm, Sonia Diaz Monsalve, Hamid Afshar Zanjani, Farzad Goli and Frank Kuan-Yu Chen

Case Study Mr. S. is 50 years old, married and father of 3 daughters. He has been suffering from chest pain-related symptoms for 5 years. Risk factors include high blood pressure, elevated blood lipid levels, obesity and smoking. His risk factors are poorly managed and he avoids doctor's visits. Four weeks ago, he suffered an acute posterior wall infarction.

K. Fritzsche (✉) · S. D. Monsalve
Department of Psychosomatic Medicine and Psychotherapy,
University Medical Center, Hauptstr. 8, 79104 Freiburg, Germany
e-mail: kurt.fritzsche@uniklinik-freiburg.de

S. D. Monsalve
e-mail: sonia.diaz-monsalve@uniklinik-freiburg.de

G. Frahm
Department of Human Sciences, Federal University of Paraná,
R. Gal. Carneiro, 460, Curitiba, PR 80060-150, Brazil
e-mail: gfrahm@uol.com.br

H. Afshar Zanjani
Department of Psychiatry, Isfahan University of Medical Sciences, Isfahan, Iran
e-mail: afshar@med.mui.ac.ir

Noor Hospital, Isfahan, Iran
e-mail: shafsharz@gmail.com

F. Goli
Department of bioenergy economy, Energy Medicine University, California, USA
e-mail: Dr.fgoli@yahoo.com

Danesh-e Tandorosti Institute, Isfahan, Iran
e-mail: info@iranianhealth.com

F. K.-Y. Chen
Division of Psychosomatic Medicine, Taipei City Psychiatric Center,
Taipei City Hospital, No. 309 Song-De Road, Taipei 11080, Taiwan
e-mail: kychen@ms4.hinet.net

K. Fritzsche et al. (eds.), *Psychosomatic Medicine*, DOI 10.1007/978-1-4614-1022-5_13,

Psychosocial anamnesis

When the patient was 4 years old, his mother was diagnosed with cancer and passed away when he was 12 years old after a long battle with the disease. The patient is still missing her to this day. The father had no emotional understanding for the boy's needs. "Performance is all that counts". In the aftermath of the myocardial infarction, the patient finds him to be ignorant and depreciative ("lazy bone!").

The patient is a trained auto mechanic. He worked extremely hard up to the point when he fell ill ("indispensable"), with little reward. He perceived the work as being menial ("slaving and sweating away").

He was regularly upset, had repeated fits of rage leading to conflicts at work and at home. He tried compensating states of intense inner tension and irritation with excessive eating and alcohol consumption.

Definition

Coronary heart disease (CHD) denotes a deficient supply of the heart with oxygen due to increasing narrowing of the coronary arteries (Angina pectoris) up to total occlusion of the vessels eliciting a coronary infarction. The consequences of tissue destruction in infarction are impairment of the cardiac pump function with heart failure and cardiac arrhythmias with sudden cardiac death.

Psychosocial problems after myocardial infarction are: destabilization of self-esteem, the fear of cardiac complications, loss of physical integrity, loss of job and decreased social status, dependence on doctors and caregivers and defense of aggressive impulses.

Relevance

The known risk factors for coronary heart disease are hypertension, elevated serum values of LDL cholesterol and triglycerides, diabetes mellitus, smoking, overweight and lack of exercise. In addition to genetic factors, psychosocial stress especially depression, in interaction with somatic risk factors, also plays a decisive role in the onset and course of coronary heart disease. The risk of heart attack can be reduced by 80 % by changing the individual lifestyle, for example by quitting smoking, healthy diet, more exercise and less stress. After myocardial infarction, 20 % of patients meet the criteria of a depressive disorder and have an elevated risk of death.

Theory

Symptoms

Emotional stress during the first several days after an acute cardiac infarction:

Anxiety

Anxiety is the most significant psychological symptom during the acute phase. Anxiety can increase to the point of panic with a sense of mortal danger. Anxiety manifests itself as a trembling voice, fearful facial expression, clingy behaviour, frequent asking of reassuring questions and suspicious controlling behaviour. Anxiety is caused by the continuing angina pectoris symptoms, menacing phantasies about the cause and consequences of the cardiac infarction, loss of control, dependence on medical devices, fear of permanent damages and impairments.

Depression

All in all, a depressed patient appears to react slower, displays a lack of interest and is often reclusive. Helplessness to the point of self-abandonment is hidden behind the silent inconspicuousness. These symptoms often go unnoticed in the hustle and bustle of acute care hospitals. In addition to an unspecific reaction to the disease, the symptoms are mainly caused by a sense of helplessness, repelled aggressive impulses such as rage and grief directed at oneself, prior professional and/or personal resentments or a depressive personality structure.

Diagnostic Categories

- Acute stress reaction (ICD-10: F43.0)
- Adjustment disorders (ICD-10: F43.2)

Frequency

Coronary heart disease is the most common cause of death in Western countries.

States of anxiety and depressive symptoms are observed in about 30 % of patients in the first days and weeks following an acute cardiac infarction.

Table 13.1 Psychosocial stress factors associated with a higher risk of coronary heart disease and heart attack

Emotional stress factors	Occupational stress factors
Negative bonding experience	Excessive willingness to work with underestimation of the demands and overestimation of one's own strength coupled with a need for importance and recognition
Problems of self-esteem	High professional demands with concurrent low control and room for decisions about the tasks to be performed and their results
Chronic partnership conflicts	High engagement with low returns in terms of pay, respect, job security and chance for advancement
Hostility	Lack of good relationships on the job
Social isolation	
Vital exhaustion	
Depression	

Onset and Course

Psychosocial Factors in Coronary Heart Disease

All of the psychosocial stress factors listed below (Table 13.1) have been found in several studies to be associated with a 2–3 times higher risk of coronary heart disease and heart attack.

Gender-Specific Aspects of Coronary Heart Disease

In women, the age of manifestation initially rises moderately after the onset of menopause, and then exponentially in the higher age groups (starting from age 75). The cardiovascular mortality is higher than in men. This is likely due to the double burden of professional and family-related stress. Additional psychosocial stress factors in women include partnership, children, grandchildren and other family-related problem areas.

Correlation Between Depression and CHD

Depression is a confirmed demonstrated risk factor for the outcome of coronary heart disease. The mortality risk was 3–4 times higher for patients with clinically relevant depression. The correlation between depression and cardiovascular disease is illustrated in Table 13.2.

Interaction of the Risk Factors

Due to an accumulation of stressful experiences in childhood rather fearful or suspicious interpretation and behaviour patterns develop. This leads to stress reactions in interpersonal relationships. A prolonged imbalance of stress systems increases

Table 13.2 Correlation between Depression and Cardiovascular Diseases

Depression		
HPA Axis[a]	Sympathovagal Dysregulation	Altered Health Behaviour
Hypercortisonemia • Elevated blood lipids • Adiposity • Insulin resistance • Diabetes mellitus	Impaired endothelial function Arrhythmias Vasoconstriction Hypertension	Noncompliance, e.g. medications Smoking Too-little exercise Unhealthy diet

[a]HPA = Hypothalamus-Pituitary-Adrenal-Axis

depressive symptoms and promotes an unhealthy disease behaviour such as smoking, unhealthy diet and physical inactivity. On the other hand, depression in turn represents a persistent internal stressor that impacts the development of coronary heart disease through activation of the immune system, of blood coagulation and changes to the vascular endothelium (Table 13.2). The interaction of these somatic and psychosocial risk factors increases tenfold the probability of dying a cardiac death at an early age.

Practice

Recognition

Although many patients experience the heart attack as occurring "out of the blue", one-quarter of the patients had uncharacteristic warning signs which, however, are usually ignored. Among these are fatigue, performance weakness, impaired concentration, dizziness, insomnia, anxiety and a feeling of being ill. These symptoms are denoted by the term "vital exhaustion".

Basic Therapeutic Attitude

The doctor obtains a better understanding of the patient's thoughts and behaviour within the scope of the **biopsychosocial anamnesis**. She/he gets to know the patient's disease concept and identifies maladaptive coping strategies. In addition to determining past psychosocial stresses, the ward physician offers regular short discussions. The doctor's continuous attention, compassion and emotional support help the patient experience a sense of equalization for narcissistic indignations and the loss of physical performance. The goal is to provide the patient with a sense of security, reduce his fears and strengthen his trust into the medical treatment.

Basic Interventions

Acute Phase

In the acute phase, the patient is in ambivalence between his wish for independence and hypochondriacal fears. The anxious side and the wish for regression are combated by a dominant and expansive manner so as not to lose "control".

Practice Tips The doctor attempts to understand and accept the patient in his emotional ambivalence, by *reflecting both sides* to him:

- "You have always been used to controlling your own life and making your own decisions. Now you are dependent on doctors, nurses and machines, and maybe for the first time in your life you are feeling something like fear and helplessness. If you wish, you can tell me more about what you are thinking and feeling."
- "How did you feel emotionally when you learned you had had a heart attack? I can imagine, and I have heard from other patients, that it was rather a shock at first."

The doctor informs the patient about the goals of treatment and the plan for treatment, as well as techniques to reduce lack of confidence and anxiety. Depending on the patient's need for information, potential causes of the heart attack may be discussed:

- "A heart attack seldom comes out of the blue. What have you had to put up with in recent months?"

Postinfarction Phase

The need for rest and the slowly-returning work capacity is experienced by many patients as passivity which is hard to bear. Their lives were formerly dictated by self-confirmation based on performance and not compatible with longer bed-rest and "coddling". Therefore, these patients soon show a tendency to take up their old life and work-style, for example with respect to smoking, diet, overtime.

Measures for prevention and treatment of coronary heart disease that address only changes in lifestyle (e.g. dietary advice, guidance on physical activity, nonsmoking training) may fall short in many cases. Rather, treating the psychological "scars" of earlier psychosocial stress should also be taken into account. In this regard, the therapeutic doctor–patient relationship offers an important field of learning in which maladaptive relationship patterns that lead to emotional distress become apparent, and may also be changed.

Antidepressant Drugs

Patients with moderate or serious depressive episodes during the acute or chronic phase of coronary heart disease benefit from SSRIs (e.g. Sertraline) and Mirtazapine.

However, the contraindications and warnings for the individual substances in connection with coronary heart disease should be taken into consideration.

Maladaptive coping strategies as denial of a heart attack are coupled with the following consequences :

- Calling the doctor too late.
- Angina pectoris symptoms are not recognized and not taken seriously.
- Prescribed bed-rest is not followed.
- Information on the onset of coronary infarction and consequential performance of later therapy and rehabilitation is selectively understood.
- The brief improvement in emotional wellbeing due to denial is purchased at the cost after 1 year of poorer compliance, more frequent rehospitalization and an increased mortality rate.

Pitfalls

- The doctor is overwhelmed by the reports about past achievements and feels that his/her offer to talk is rejected. However, the "stories" often mask indications of severe anxiety, negative relationship experiences and relationship desires.
- Some patients negate the threat of their physical health condition with the heart disease. The patient comes across as emotionally unfazed, is rigid and refuses to cooperate. The doctor understands that the denial may represent a protection against the unbearable feelings of destruction and social isolation.

Cooperation

The need for psychotherapeutic support exists in 20 % of patients both in the acute hospitalization and in outpatient or in-hospital rehabilitation.

The following treatment measures have proven beneficial:

- Cognitive-behavioural training programmes to reduce stress and promote health-conscious behaviour, with the aim of influencing cardiovascular risk factors.
- Psychotherapeutic modification of coronary-endangering behavioural or personality characteristics, such as suppressed anger, social withdrawal.
- Psychotherapeutic and psychopharmacological treatment of depression.

Meta-analyses show that short-term psychotherapeutic interventions reduce psychosocial stress and lead to a significant improvement of the psychological wellbeing and quality of life. The interventions normalized the heart rate, reduced cholesterol levels and reduced the risk of cardiac events and cardiac mortality (Linden et al. 2007).

Cultural Aspects

Iran

In Persian medical system heart is regarded to be the central organ to control the emotions and the location of life's energy. Because of its very tangible and instant responses to the mental and the physical alternations, traditionally it has been recognized as mind–body connection and whole body organizer (see also the cultural aspects of the chapters anxiety and somatoform disorders). Disorders of heart function therefore receive special attention. An irregular heartbeat may indicate personal emotional issues or problems in interpersonal relationships. The symptom attributions of patients with respect to cardiac symptoms include a long list of biopsychosocial causes (Good 1977): sadness, anxiety, thoughts of death, debt, poverty, conflicts, family problems and diseases, specific problems in everyday life, pregnancy, childbirth, unhappy marriage and many somatic attributions, such as anaemia, low blood pressure, vitamin deficiency.

Knowing music is one the basic skills of healers because they should distinguish about 50 normal and abnormal pulses as Avicenna explained in *canon* and *resalat fi nabz* (Morewedge 1973). Various musical modalities of pulse were explored as: rhythm, frequency, range, tension, colour and harmony and evidently, in such a medical model music therapy would have very important role in reorganizing the both, mental and physical disharmonies. Otherwise, monitoring of pulse during the traditional music therapy session was the main cue for adjustment of music to obtain ultimate psychosomatic balance.

Normal variations of pulse, present the nature and personality of the patient and abnormal rhythms signify the disorders of body–mind. For example, as a normal variation, a humid temper heart has a soft pulsation, and mild to moderate impulsivity and labile mood. But excessive humid temperament of heart is characterized by very soft pulse and unstable mood and affect, and such a heart is prone to infection fevers. So pulse in this health system is supposed as a polyphonic symphony that structural and functional characteristics of a human organism, and also mental and physical modes are manifested through.

Taiwan

A study over the beliefs about the heart disease of the patients with coronary artery diseases (CAD) showed that the Taiwanese patients had more misconceived and maladaptive beliefs, in comparison to their British counterparts (Lin et al. 2008). Relatively lower prevalence rate of CAD in Taiwan, less well-developed service for CAD patients and the influence of the Chinese culture may account for the difference. A Canadian study revealed a similar finding: New immigrants from Chinese societies lack the awareness of heart disease and stroke (Chow et al. 2008).

Latin America

Latin American Continent is facing a growth of ageing population, as well as a significant boost in urban population, which has increased poverty, sedentarism and obesity. This has been causing health deterioration in general, with significant increase of coronary heart disease. Research studies show increases in hypertension, hyperglycemia and high levels of cholesterol. Coronary heart disease has been causing the highest mortality rates, as high as 34 % or more in the overall American countries; the USA, for example, has been making attempts to bring CHD under control since 1960.

Health authorities have been taking some prevention actions to face the increase of coronary heart disease, which have been mostly based on programmes providing orientation for the development of healthy living habit, as well as some follow-up home visits for the most affected ones. Unfortunately, despite efforts and optimism of health authorities, research findings have brought to light that measures taken so far have shown no significant changes in life style of the population submitted to the provided general educational procedures. Coronary heart disease continues to increase. As regards to prevention and treatment, finding evidenced it to be still precarious, mostly amongst those who rely on the government free health care system, whilst the ones who pay private health care are better looked after.

References

Chow CM, Chu JW, Tu JV, Moe GW. Lack of awareness of heart disease and stroke among Chinese Canadians: results of a pilot study of the Chinese Canadian Cardiovascular Health Project. Can J Cardiol. 2008;24(8):623–8.

Good BJ. The heart of what's the matter: The semantics of illness in Iran. Cult Med Psychiat. 1977;1:25–58.

Lin YP, Furze G, Spilsbury K, Lewin RJP. Misconceived and maladaptive beliefs about heart disease: a comparison between Taiwan and Britain. J Clin Nurs. 2008;18:46–55.

Linden W, Phillips MJ, Leclerc J. Psychological treatment of cardiac patients: a meta-analysis. Eur Heart J. 2007;28:2972–84.

Morewedge P. Danishnama-i 'ala'i (The Book of Scientific Knowledge). The Metaphysics of Avicenna. London: Routledge and Kegan Paul; 1973.

Chapter 14
Acute and Posttraumatic Stress Disorder (PTSD)

Kurt Fritzsche, Catherine Abbo, Gertrud Frahm, Sonia Diaz Monsalve and Frank Kuan-Yu Chen

Case Study A 45-year-old ENT physician was critically injured by a drunken 52-year-old patient with multiple stab wounds in the abdomen. This followed a verbal dispute from the patient's perspective, due to unsatisfactory treatment outcome. The doctor was treated at the hospital emergency room and then transferred to a normal ward. In the following days he developed anxiety in enclosed spaces, seemed mostly irritable and complaint of insomnia and restlessness. Upon questioning, he told about very frightening dreams that were directly or indirectly related to his experience of violence. He then woke up drenched in sweat and had trouble to get his bearings. Initially, he avoided to talk about these experiences and his mental condition. Only by careful inquiries of the ward physician it was possible to gather the full extent of the acute trauma.

(continued)

K. Fritzsche (✉) · S. D. Monsalve
Department of Psychosomatic Medicine and Psychotherapy, University Medical Center, Hauptstr. 8, 79104 Freiburg, Germany
e-mail: kurt.fritzsche@uniklinik-freiburg.de

S. D. Monsalve
e-mail: sonia.diaz-monsalve@uniklinik-freiburg.de

C. Abbo
Department of Psychiatry, Makerere University College of Health Sciences and Mulago National Referral and Teaching Hospital, Mulago Hill Road, 7072 Kampala, Uganda
e-mail: cathyabbo@chs.mak.ac.ug, cathya180@gmail.com

G. Frahm
Department of Human Sciences, Federal University of Paraná, R. Gal. Carneiro, 460, Curitiba, PR 80060-150, Brazil
e-mail: gfrahm@uol.com.br

F. K.-Y. Chen
Division of Psychosomatic Medicine, Taipei City Psychiatric Center, Taipei City Hospital, No. 309 Song-De Road, Taipei 11080, Taiwan
e-mail: kychen@ms4.hinet.net

K. Fritzsche et al. (eds.), *Psychosomatic Medicine,* DOI 10.1007/978-1-4614-1022-5_14,

Definition

Psychological trauma is defined as the result of a momentary or prolonged stressful event that is beyond normal human experience and that would be stressful for anyone. The defining characteristic is the large discrepancy between external threats and the available coping skills.

A traumatic event meets the following criteria:

- The person was a victim or witness of an event in which one's own life or the lives of others were threatened or as a result had a serious injury, for example, natural disaster, war, traffic accident, diagnosis of a terminal illness, stay in intensive care, terrorism, rape and violent crime.
- The reaction of the person concerned involves feelings of intense fear, helplessness and horror.
- Due to the traumatic experience, the confidence in oneself and others is shaken fundamentally.

Another classification is often linked to the duration of the potentially traumatic event. Traumatisation, which was caused by a rather short and single event (e.g. serious accident or sexual abuse in adulthood) is referred to as Type I trauma, and a longer lasting and repeated trauma (repeated physical and sexual abuse in childhood) as Type II trauma. In Type I trauma, usually there are very clear, vivid memories of the event and there is a classic picture of posttraumatic stress disorder (PTSD), whereas, in Type II trauma often there are only diffuse, little clear recollections. Here, very different comorbid mental disorders (e.g. anxiety, depression, physical symptoms and eating disorders) may occur.

Relevance

It is assumed that traumatic experiences which have not been processed to a sufficient extent and integrated are a reason for numerous physical and psychological complaints, which arise in primary care. A traumatisation increases the likelihood of developing other mental illnesses such as depression, anxiety disorders, somatoform disorders and drug and substance abuse. Identifying trauma in time and providing necessary care will shorten the suffering and prevent the chronicity of symptoms.

Theory

Symptoms

One can distinguish three groups of symptoms of PTSD.

Intrusions

Obsessive intrusive images such as nightmares, flashbacks or other sensations such as noise and strong sense of smell that directly emerge from the triggering event (accident, robbery etc.) are difficult to access by the voluntary control of the person concerned (*intrusion symptoms*).

Hyperarousal

Severe irritability, sleep disturbances, lack of concentration and overall significantly reduced physical and mental stamina.

Avoidance

Places and situations that are mentally and emotionally related to the traumatic experience are avoided. The feelings are superficial.

Other consequential symptoms of PTSD include sense of shame and guilt, identification with the aggressor, dissociation, self-harming and violence against others.

The long-term effects of PTSD are:

- Lasting personality changes such as hostility, distrust, withdrawal, chronic emptiness and feelings of alienation (Diagnosis F 62.0)
- Muscle or joint pain due to continuous strain of the deep structure of the muscles as a result of the interrupted, quasi-frozen fight or flight reactions in the acute phase of trauma stored in the body memory
- Lower abdominal pain after sexual intercourse as a result of sexual trauma

Diagnostic Categories

Acute Stress Disorder (ICD-10: F43.0)

This is a temporary disorder of an otherwise mentally stable person following an extraordinary physical and/or emotional stress, which subsides within 4 weeks after the trauma. The symptoms include a shock reaction, feeling of absence, numbness and disorientation, as well as hyperactivity and autonomic arousal. These are adequate emotional and physical ways of reacting to heavy stress.

Adjustment Disorder (ICD-10: F43.2)

The psychological responses, mostly in the form of depressive or anxious symptoms may last several months up to half a year. There are patients who actively deal with the trauma and related psychological and physical symptoms, and others who try to numb themselves with alcohol or tranquilizers.

Posttraumatic Stress Disorder: PTSD (ICD-10: F43.1)

The symptoms occur within few weeks to 6 months (acute PTSD), or 6 months and later (delayed-onset PTSD) after the traumatic event. The symptoms last for more than a month. The person concerned is affected psychologically and socially.

Lasting Personality Change After Extreme Stress (ICD-10: F62.0)

The disorder is characterized by a hostile or distrustful attitude towards the world, a feeling of alienation, feelings of emptiness or hopelessness and a chronic feeling of tension. Posttraumatic stress disorder may have preceded this type of personality change.

Outlook DSM-V: Complex Trauma

Based on field investigations initiated by the DSM-working group of the APA, a more complex disease pattern has been identified that arises not only in the wake of severe trauma such as physical or sexual abuse experiences, but also of war and torture experiences or abductions and was conceptualized as ('Disorder of Extreme Stress Not Otherwise Specified' (DESNOS), Appendix DSM-IV). This category is to be redrafted and incorporated in the next revision of the DSM (Version V) as 'Complex Post Traumatic Stress Disorder'.

Frequency

Depending on the age of those affected, the lifetime prevalence of PTSD is 1.1 and 2.9 % (Wittchen et al. 2011). Substantially higher is the probability of the occurrence of less pronounced disorders. Women are affected twice as often as men. The occurrence of PTSD depends on the kind of trauma: Trauma due to violation: PTSD prevalence of 50 %, 25 % due to other violent felony, 20 % due to war victims. Trauma due to serious, life-threatening illness, e.g. cancer: PTSD prevalence of 15 %. Trauma due to intensive-medical measures, e.g. polytrauma: PTSD prevalence of 5 %. Trauma due to accident, e.g. traffic accident: PTSD prevalence of 18 % (Kessler et al. 1995).

Onset

The *acute phase,* also referred to as shock phase lasts up to 1 week.

The following weeks are characterized by the attempt to live a normal life again and to process and integrate the trauma as an extreme experience. During this phase, which is referred to as the *impact phase,* not only a whole range of mental health symptoms—mainly anxiety and avoidance—may occur, but also depressive symptoms with increasing duration of exposure. This phase can last several months to half a year. Then, the memories of the trauma slowly fade and the symptoms subside (*recovery phase*). In about one-third of all patients, *chronification* must be expected.

Practice

Acute Trauma

Basic Therapeutic Attitude

Early interventions aim for basal *calming, safety* and *stabilisation*. They should offer patients a *safe space with clear boundaries*. They should be directed *less towards emotions,* but primarily to *relaxation* and a *reduction* of the psychophysiological *stress symptoms*. The doctor's speech should be simple, slow, repetitious, objective and transparent.

Basic Interventions

The five essentials elements of trauma treatment are *hope,* a sense of *safety, calming,* a sense of *self- and community-efficiency* and *connectedness* (Hobfoll et al. 2007). These principles can already be applied during the first 4 weeks.

A Safe Place

The most important thing in an acute crisis situation is to create a safe place where the arousal of the patient can subside and he is back to himself.

Flashback management and dissociation stop. When patients are in a distressing dissociative state, it may be therapeutically necessary to help them to get out of this condition, so that they can reorient again in reality.

- Address the patient sternly, loudly, if necessary, give direction to the reality in the here and now.
  'Mrs. A, are you still here? Look around: You are safe!'
- Ask the patient to look around the room and to name five objects that he/she can see.
- You can hand the patient an ice cube or a hedgehog ball in order to draw attention to the sensory stimulus, even strong scents with a stimulating effect may be helpful.

Anamnesis and Resources Exploration

Case Study (Continued) In our case study also, the ward physician initially creates an undisturbed atmosphere for talking. Outside the door she hangs a sign reading, 'do not disturb'. Only when the patient has found a relaxed sitting position, she asks the patient about his present condition and, in terms of a narrative interviewing, she provides room for his experience. Possible topics of conversation can be found under 'Practical tip'.

(continued)

Practical Tip Brief resource-oriented anamnesis

- Current symptoms
- Event only in keywords: no invasive questions, no details, do not ask about emotions, keep everything superficial and at a distance
- Earlier traumatisations and coping with them (trauma profile)
- Respect or support avoidances

Explore resources

- 'What in your life has been helpful in difficult situations to calm down and to feel safe'? (make the patient tell concrete situations in more detail, if possible)
- 'What is benefitting you in your life today'? (anything that gives pleasure, is important and is benefitting in more detail)
- 'What has earlier brought comfort and was helpful'?

Always couple all associations with the traumatic event back to positive resources

'. . . and you did the best thing in the situation. . . and you survived. . .'

Psychoeducation

Case Study (Continued) In another consultation, the ward physician provides the patient with information about the relationship between his acute trauma and his current thoughts, feelings, physical sensations and behavioural impulses. She advises what measures have proven to be helpful for emotional stability. Examples can be found under 'Practical tip'.

Practical Tip Providing information about trauma

- Simple models in simple, slow language, oriented to information already obtained from the patient: The current symptoms and state are the normal reaction to an abnormal, traumatic event/extreme stress. Most people would react this way. 'The nervous system is flooded with stress hormones by

such an event and needs time and a quiet environment to deal with the trauma/extreme stress with its own inherent self-healing powers'.
'You can do something'—mediation of whole and self-efficiency
- Keep all stimulation and stressful things and inputs at a distance, watch little TV, do not read newspapers
- Easily manageable diversion
- Emotional and practical support from important and close people
- Permission: talk when, about what, with whom, how long; you may or even must say *no*
- Provide safety and protection

Daily agenda and helpful activities
- Discuss and support structures agenda
- Pick up on all helpful habits and daily rituals which were pleasant, relaxing and comforting before and after the trauma
- Try everything of these that still works and do it more often
- Reactivate the social network in everyday life

Interventions on an Imaginative Level

Whenever traumatic or terrifying material threatens to flood the patient, ask them to lock these images and ideas in an imaginary vault or safe, where they will be stored until a sufficient stabilisation allows for their processing. In this exercise, defence mechanisms of denial and repression are specifically supported.

Psychopharmaceutical Treatment

In higher degrees of traumatisation, insomnia should be treated by Zopiclon 7.5 mg or Mirtazapin 15 mg at night. In cases of moderate or severe depression, selective serotonin reuptake inhibitors (SSRI) are necessary.

Cave: Benzodiazepines promote fixation of traumatic memories and should therefore be very limited in use.

Up to 4 Weeks After Psychotrauma

- Fulfilment of primary needs
- Create and mediate physical safety
- Practical and emotional support
- Psychoeducation/ information
- Stabilisation, medications (in higher degrees of traumatisation)
- 'watchful waiting' (in milder traumatisation)

Pitfalls

- Especially in temporal proximity to the event, there is the increased risk of *re-traumatisation* through flashback-like reliving of the traumatic situation with the consequence of a renewed mental instability. Therefore, direct or repeated inquiries with respect to the traumatic situation must be avoided in order not to jeopardise the stabilisation that has occurred already.
- On the other hand, there is the risk that the treating physician supports the avoidance behaviour of the patient beyond the period necessary. This prevents the integration of the traumatic experience in the patient's personality, a mental splitting is looming.
- Helpers in a potentially traumatic situation must protect themselves also. The probability of occurrence of secondary traumatisations is relatively high.
- Relaxation exercises, e.g. autogenous training can promote regression and should not be used.

Posttraumatic Stress Disorder (PTSD)

PTSD is diagnosed if the symptoms do not regress, and present over a period of 4 weeks still in onerous form. The onset of symptoms can be delayed, where, after the traumatic event, initially there is symptom-free time. The aim here is coping with what has been experienced by integration and compensation of the traumatic experiences.

Case study 60-year-old Ms. Hill presents to the family doctor. In her second marriage, she has been married for 20 years, has 2 children and 2 grandchildren. She lives with her husband in a small town near the doctor's office. She is treated by the family doctor for her high blood pressure and joint pain in the hands, which becomes increasingly more painful. Currently, after not having visited the doctor's office for a very long time, the patient attends an appointment because of insomnia and inner tension. When asked by the doctor about stressful events in the near and far past, Ms. Hill reported a car accident two and a half years ago, in which the 4-year-old grandchild died. Her husband momentarily nodded off, went off the road and the car flipped over. While she herself suffered only a few bruises, the granddaughter passed away from internal bleeding. Since then, the husband has become a mere shadow of his former self. Her first husband also died in a car accident at the beginning of her first marriage.

(continued)

Recognition

For patients who seek the doctor's help for not only nonspecific symptoms such as insomnia, tachycardia, sweating, tension, irritability, depressed mood, but also alcohol and drug abuse, and report interpersonal and professional conflicts, one should always consider the possibility of PTSD. Especially, when the psychological reaction to an acute event, such as a minor accident, death of a distant relative appears seemingly inadequate, one should always ask cautiously (risk of re-traumatisation) about an accident or other violent actions in the patient's history. Based on the description of the patient, the doctor will then decide the phase (acute phase, the impact phase or chronic phase) in which the patient is.

Case Study (Continued) Ms. Hill reports sleep disturbances and inner tension. Upon sympathetic enquiry of the doctor she also mentions that she sometimes relives the accident like in a movie, especially when driving on a country road. Then, she starts sweating, becomes dizzy, and her heart races. She no longer can think clearly and cannot stop the movie. Then she feels stunned, not knowing what to do with herself. In the evening or at night, she dreams about the accident, and often wakes up sweating. She also shows strong reactions when seeing newspaper articles about accidents or when others by chance talk about minor accidents. Overall, she is more restless, more irritable and can no longer focus. In everyday situations, pictures of the accident come over her uncontrollably. While reporting her experiences to the doctor, the patient appears very tense, speaks hesitantly, does not look at the doctor rather looks restlessly back and forth in the room.

Based on the medical history and current symptoms, the doctor can make a diagnosis of PTSD, and thereby, timely initiate an important change in the direction of a targeted psychotherapy.

Cooperation

Trauma detective work has the objective to make the traumatic experiences re-liveable in order to be able to integrate them into the overall personality. Trauma detective work is subject to the following conditions:

- Adequate stabilisation of the patient, no acute psychopathology in need of psychiatric treatment
- Sufficient trauma-specific skills of the therapist, enough experience with trauma exposure
- No offender contact whatsoever
- No severe dissociative states, from risk of severe mental decompensation to suicidality in the emergence of traumatic memories

Example of Detective Trauma Work Trauma exposition (remembrance)

- As an introduction, reactivating self-calming and positive inner images (safe place, helpers inside)
- Divide trauma processing into individual steps, schedule intervals for stabilisation
- Techniques: screen technology, eye movement desensitization and reprocessing (EDMR), a bilateral stimulation of both hemispheres of the brain in the form of auditory or tactile stimulation

Cultural Aspects

Africa

It is necessary for primary health care workers to gain an understanding of religious and spiritual healing and its role in healing patients with trauma. Below are detailed aspects from Africa with an example from the Acholi people of Northern Uganda.

Case Study 'Acholi people in Northern Uganda' The Acholi people in Northern Uganda have constructive and dynamic approach to the task of dealing with traumatic experiences of the Lord's Resistance Army returnees for the purposes of reintegration in the community. The returnees, especially children experience bad dreams and nightmares. According to the Acholi people, the dreams and the nightmares are bad spirits that disturb the children and this must be dealt with accordingly. Communities have a number of rituals, which can rid the child of the cen and restore peace to him or her. These ceremonies are intertwined with:

- The language of forgiveness
- Healing
- Restoration

One specific ritual, referred to locally as 'the breaking of eggs' is utilised to acknowledge children's physical and spiritual absence, return and cleansing and to make them a member of the family. In this ceremony the child walks on a path and is required to step on and break some eggs. Towards the end of the ceremony, the child walks through the door of the house, and then water is poured over his or her head. By the time the child has completed the ritual process, the broken eggs are left behind and the child emerges as cleansed.

The role of religion and spirituality in healing the emotional and psychological effects of psychotrauma is two-folds:

1. To restore spiritual equilibrium shuttered by the effects of trauma on the individual, family and community

2. To tap into the positive aspects of religious and spiritual coping to facilitate emotional and psychological healing of the effects of trauma

Primary health care workers' role is to facilitate these two processes in the clients who are spiritually oriented be it traditional African religion or any other, and who may be going through an existential crisis of a spiritual nature. There is a need to be sensitive to cues about the client's spiritual orientation as they talk about their trauma story. It should be remembered that many persons from the African sociocultural contexts have dual religious inclinations, that is inclinations that have elements of both traditional African religious practice and Judeo-Christian and Islamic influences.

How Health Workers May Facilitate Religious/Spiritual Healing

Traumatised patients need/want: answers, justice, relief from negative emotions, to get on with their lives. Most Africans are religious and have religious identities something that can be harnessed to help them effectively deal with emotional and psychological effects of trauma. Health worker can facilitate religious and spiritual healing through the following:

- Assessing the religious and spiritual identity and needs of their clients. Using a standardized tool to do this (see note above) and refer those who require and will benefit from religious/spiritual healing.
- Need to know the 'good' religious/spiritual healing resources in their community. Ideally should have formal contact with these practices where to refer their clients.

Fica Peel—A Tool for Assessing Religious/Spiritual Identity and Needs of Trauma Clients

- How important is *faith* in your daily life?
- How do your beliefs *influence* daily life?
- Are you a member of a religious *community* and how can they help you?
- How would you like your spiritual needs to be *addressed* in your treatment?
- All your clients should have a *psychiatric* evaluation before referring them for religious/spiritual healing.
- Get the client's and importantly others' spiritual *explanations* for the trauma, e.g. if is it due to a curse etc.
- Is the client's *experience* in keeping with those of immediate significant others and with cultural and religious beliefs of that community.
- Mental health workers need to *liaise* and appreciate the role of religious/spiritual healers in trauma management.

Taiwan

Due to the culture stressing obedience from children, corporeal punishment is well accepted and prevalent in Taiwan and other Chinese societies. A study showed that about one-third of children in Taiwan experienced physical violence in their lives, a rate much higher than that of Western societies. The prevalence of PTSD related to physical abuse is also higher, about 13.6 % of the maltreated children (Chou et al. 2011).

Regarding the PTSD related to natural disasters in Taiwan, mainly typhoons and earthquakes, many religious groups, such as Tzu-Chi foundation (Buddhist), Chinese Christian Relief Association, Presbyterian Church in Taiwan and so on, provided many relief actions but there is still no published scientific study to follow the effects of these relief actions.

Latin American

Armed conflict in Colombia has resulted in the displacement of an estimated 4.5 million people, or about 10 % of the Colombian population. Hundreds of thousands of Colombians are exposed to violence and forced displacement annually. PTSD occurs frequently but is not detected or treated early. This severe problem has been highlighted in the study by Richards et al. using survey methods to assess levels of PTSD in the city of Medellin in a sample of 109 internally displaced adults. A large proportion of respondents showed clinically significant PTSD (88 %). Focus group findings suggested that participants were interested in specialised psychological treatments as well as broader psychosocial interventions to treat the consequences of exposure to violence and forced displacement (Richards et al. 2011).

References

Chou CY, Su YJ, Wu HM, Chen SH. Child physical abuse and the related PTSD in Taiwan: The role of Chinese cultural background and victims' subjective reactions. Child Abuse Neglect. 2011;35:58–68.

Hobfoll SE, Watson P, Bell CC, Bryant RA, Brymer MJ, Friedman MJ, et al. Five essential elements of immediate and mid-term mass trauma intervention: empirical evidence. Psychiatry. 2007;70:283–315.

Kessler RC, Sonnega A, Bromet E, Hughes M, Nelson CB. Posttraumatic stress disorder in the National Comorbidity Survey. Arch Gen Psychiatry. 1995;52(12):1048–60.

Richards A, Ospina-Duque J, Barrera-Valencia M, Escobar-Rincón J, Ardila-Gutiérrez M, Metzler T, et al. Posttraumatic stress disorder, anxiety and depression symptoms, and psychosocial treatment needs in Colombians internally displaced by armed conflict: a mixed-method evaluation. Psychol Trauma. 2011;3(4):384–93.

Wittchen HU, Jacobi F, Rehm J, Gustavsson A, Svensson M, Jönsson B, et al. The size and burden of mental disorders and other disorders of the brain in Europe 2010. Eur Neuropsychopharmacol. 2011;21:655–79.

Chapter 15
Addiction

Kurt Fritzsche, Axel Schweickhardt, Catherine Abbo, Gertrud Frahm, Sonia Diaz Monsalve, Frank Kuan-Yu Chen, Kim Viet Nguyen and Van Tuan Nguyen

Case Study An approximately 40-year-old man visits the family practitioner because of recurrent nausea and pressure symptoms in the upper abdomen. Based on the initial examinations, the family physician diagnoses gastritis;

K. Fritzsche (✉) · S. D. Monsalve
Department of Psychosomatic Medicine and Psychotherapy,
University Medical Center, Hauptstr. 8, 79104 Freiburg, Germany
e-mail: kurt.fritzsche@uniklinik-freiburg.de

S. D. Monsalve
e-mail: sonia.diaz-monsalve@uniklinik-freiburg.de

A. Schweickhardt
Potenziale GmbH Business Consultants, Peyerstr. 34,
90429 Nuremberg, Germany
e-mail: Schweickhardt@potenziale.biz

C. Abbo
Department of Psychiatry, Makerere University College of Health Sciences and Mulago National Referral and Teaching Hospital, Mulago Hill Road, Kampala 7072, Uganda
e-mail: cathyabbo@chs.mak.ac.ug, cathya180@gmail.com

G. Frahm
Department of Human Sciences, Federal University of Paraná,
R. Gal. Carneiro, 460, Curitiba, PR 80060-150, Brazil
e-mail: gfrahm@uol.com.br

F. K.-Y. Chen
Division of Psychosomatic Medicine, Taipei City Psychiatric Center,
Taipei City Hospital, No. 309 Song-De Road, Taipei 11080, Taiwan
e-mail: kychen@ms4.hinet.net

K. V. Nguyen · V. T. Nguyen
Department of Psychiatry, Hanoi Medical University,
No. 1, Ton That Tung Street, Dong Da District, Hanoi, Vietnam
e-mail: drnkimviet@yahoo.com

National Institute of Mental Health, Bach Mai Hospital
No. 78, Giai Phong Road, Dong Da District, Hanoi, Vietnam

V. T. Nguyen
e-mail: nvtuannimhvn@hmu.edu.vn

K. Fritzsche et al. (eds.), *Psychosomatic Medicine*, DOI 10.1007/978-1-4614-1022-5_15,

however, he harbours the suspicion of a possible alcohol dependence of the patient. Upon further inquiries, the patient tells about consuming daily three to four bottles of beer, sometimes also hard liquors. He does it to relax better and to fall asleep faster. At the workplace, he was currently under a lot of pressure, sometimes fearing to lose his job. At weekends, it is possible that the patient consumes up to half a bottle of cognac by himself. He tolerates this well and is not hung over the following day—he appears almost proud of it.

Definition

The World Health Organization (WHO) defines dependence as an insurmountable craving for a particular substance or a particular behaviour that can no longer be controlled and is dominating. The basis of dependence is the desire to experience the psychological effects of the addictive substance, increasingly, also the need to avoid unpleasant consequences of its absence (withdrawal symptoms such as restlessness, insomnia, headaches, anxiety, sweating). It leads to an increased tolerance and sometimes to a physical withdrawal syndrome. During the course, the supply and consumption of the respective substances can develop into a life-determining matter. There is a distinction between *dependence syndrome* and *harmful use*. The latter refers to—as a weaker variant of the abuse behaviour—a consumption having demonstrably a harmful effect (physically or mentally), without the presence of any dependence.

Relevance

A vast majority of alcohol-dependent patients can be found in general hospitals and private practices. Only a minority speaks openly with a general practitioner about their problems. On the other hand, even physicians have difficulty recognizing an addiction, to confront the patient with it and to offer treatment options. The open dialogue is made more difficult because many patients present with functional disorders or symptoms of pain; such complaints are at the forefront and an addiction is denied and trivialized.

Theory

Symptoms

The main symptoms of addiction are:

- Loss of control
- Withdrawal syndrome

- Development of tolerance

Indirect clinical evidence for alcohol dependence includes a reduced general state of health, mental disorders such as anxiety, poor concentration, changes in appetite, sleep patterns and sexual functions. Also, hypertension, supraventricular arrhythmias, increased sweating, a slightly enlarged liver and tenderness in the epigastrium is seen. Twenty percent of the patients show signs of polyneuropathy.

Drug-dependent patients suffer from many symptoms that are usually experienced through the body such as general depression, rapid fatigability, decreasing performance, sleep disturbances, headache, body aches, muscle pain, tension, anxiety and other somatoform disorders.

Diagnostic Categories

- Acute intoxication (ICD-10: by alcohol F10.0 and other psychoactive substances F11.0–F19.0)
- Harmful use (ICD-10: by alcohol F10.1 and other psychoactive substances F11.1–F19.1)
- Dependence syndrome (ICD-10: chronic alcoholism F10.2 or other psychoactive substances: F11.2–F19.2)

Frequency

Alcohol dependence and opioid and cannabis dependence rank together as the fourth most frequent group of mental disorders. The lifetime prevalence of alcohol dependence in Europe is about 3.4 % (Wittchen et al. 2011).

Onset

Regarding the development of dependence, a multicausal model is used, in which there are interactions of genetic predisposition, personality structure, drug and social environment (family, social class, occupation, cultural influences).

Practical Implications

Recognition

According to ICD-10, the diagnosis 'dependence' can be made, if at some point during the last year, three or more of the following criteria were simultaneously present:

- A strong desire or sense of compulsion to take the substance
- Difficulties in controlling substance-taking behaviour in terms of its onset, termination or levels of use
- A physiological withdrawal state when substance use has ceased or has been reduced, as evidenced by: the characteristic withdrawal syndrome for the substance, or the use of the same (or closely related) substance with the intention of relieving or avoiding withdrawal symptoms
- Evidence of tolerance, such that increased doses of the psychoactive substance are required in order to achieve effects originally produced by lower doses (clear examples of this are found in alcohol- and opiate-dependent individuals who may take daily doses sufficient to incapacitate or kill non-tolerant users)
- Progressive neglect of alternative pleasures or interests because of psychoactive substance use, increased amount of time necessary to obtain or take the substance or to recover from its effects
- Persisting with substance use despite clear evidence of overtly harmful consequences, such as harm to the liver through excessive drinking, depressive mood states consequent to periods of heavy substance use, or drug-related impairment of cognitive functioning; efforts should be made to determine that the user was actually, or could be expected to be, aware of the nature and extent of the harm

Indirect evidence of alcohol dependence may be obtained from an increase in the typical laboratory parameters such as gamma-GT, transaminases, mean erythrocyte cell volume (MCV) and increased carbohydrate-deficient transferrin (CDT).

These indirect methods are tempting to 'condemn' patients with so-called objective evidence. The doctor runs the risk to strengthen the defence mechanisms of the patient and to provoke a loss of contact. The best pathway to diagnosis and timely detection of an addiction problem is a dialogue with the person. If the patient does not feel immediately condemned as an addict/alcoholic, an open and informative discussion may develop.

Practical Tip 'AUDIT (alcohol use disorders identification test)'

The AUDIT questionnaire was developed on behalf of the WHO, which also recommends it. It consists of a total of ten questions that will be answered in each case on a five-point scale. The specified number of points for each question are added for a total score. The minimum score is 0, the maximum is 40. *A score of 8 or higher indicates dangerous and harmful alcohol consumption.* In women and in men over 65 years of age, it is recommended to set the limit at 7 points.

Sample questions:

- How often do you drink alcohol?
- How often have you noticed last year that you have been drinking more than you actually wanted?
- How often have you felt guilty in the past year or felt bad about your alcohol consumption?

The entire test is available online.

Table 15.1 Characteristics of motivational interviewing

Show and express empathy: This promotes acceptance and facilitates change.
Promote the perception of discrepancies and willingness to change: The patient himself/herself should provide the arguments for change.
Avoid arguments: Neither blame nor labels are constructive. Allegations generate only resistance.
Go along with the resistance of the patient: Accept the resistance of the patient to handle his/her inner conflicts.
Build confidence in self-efficacy: The patient is responsible for the decision to change and its implementation.

The diagnosis of drug dependence is complicated by the fact that patients hide the symptoms—out of shame or fear of no longer getting prescriptions for the addictive drugs. Evidence for dependence may be obtained from the following:

- Patient's resistance against attempts to discontinue the drug
- Prescription forgeries and losses
- Obtaining drugs from other doctors
- Unauthorized dose increases
- Improper use in psychological stress and to relax

Basic Therapeutic Attitude

As a basic attitude towards addicted patients, it is advised to rely on the characteristics of motivational interviewing (Miller and Rollnick 1991), which are summarized in Table 15.1.

Basic Interventions

The task of physicians in independent practices and hospitals is to provide the patient an insight into the disease and to motivate him/her for the withdrawal treatment and the subsequent detoxification treatment. Four stages of readiness to change can be distinguished (Prochaska and DiClemente 1986):

Stage 1: From Precontemplation to Contemplation

Case Study 'Asking about consumption behaviour'

Doctor: I've now completed my examination and I can say that I am presuming gastritis.

Patient: I am sure there is treatment available for it.

Doctor: Yes, there is. I would like to talk to you about possible maintaining factors and about your health behaviour. For example, do you consume alcohol and nicotine?

Patient: I quit smoking 7 years ago, from one day to the next. It was not a problem at all.

Doctor: And Alcohol?

Patient: Yes, I drink now and then. But that's normal.

Doctor: A lot of people drink regularly, that's true. How much do you consume?

Patient: About three to four beers in the evening. You have to understand! After work, I am finished. Currently, we are under a lot of pressure, and I'm a little worried of losing my job.

Doctor: That is, you drink to be able to relax better.

Patient: Yes, then I sleep wonderfully.

Doctor: What's the maximum that you can drink on an evening?

Patient: Well, at the weekend I had half a bottle of cognac. But I don't feel much, I'm not really drunk.

Doctor: And the next day?

Patient: I feel good, no problem. I can tolerate quite a bit.

Doctor: Have you thought about reducing your alcohol consumption?

Patient: Hmm. . . my wife keeps making comments.

The diagnosis of alcohol dependence is clearly communicated to the patient without demonization.

Case Study 'Communicating the diagnosis of addiction'

Doctor: After all that you've told me, and together with the results of the blood test, my diagnosis at this stage would be 'alcohol dependence'.

Patient: Oh, come on! What are you telling me?

Doctor: I can understand your reaction. It sounds like condemnation. But that's not what it is about. It's about me telling very clearly what my findings are.

(Pause)

Patient: Yes, what do we do now?

Doctor: That's the right question. What does the diagnosis imply in terms of changes?

Patient: Less drinking, I can see that, okay.

Doctor: This is also very important to recognize. Alcohol dependence is a disease and not a character flaw. And I advise you very clearly to avoid alcohol completely in the future.

Patient: What do you mean, completely? How can I possibly do that?

Stage 2: From Contemplation Towards Action

Building motivation includes the identification of discrepancies in behaviour and raising awareness of the patient, addressing his/her ambivalent stance on abstinence and coming jointly to a decision.

The patient experiences the dependence in an ambivalent manner: On one hand, he/she realises that it has assumed the form of a disease and that he/she must do something about it. On the other hand, it is the nature of addiction, to protect oneself from unbearable feelings, to balance insurmountable tensions and to create wellbeing. The patient cannot imagine having to give up the comforting companion. The result is a mixture of guilt, fear and servility. Patients develop avoidance strategies regarding a detoxification treatment. This explains why they seem to listen to the consultation patiently and attentively, but internally have long since zoned out. The doctor feels this ambivalence, and should pick it up.

Case Study 'Promotion of readiness for change'

Patient: Never drinking again, right? I don't think I can do this.

Doctor: Here, I am more confident than you! If you think about smoking, you were able to do that! I think that you could easily succeed to quit drinking alcohol also.

Patient: You may be right, indeed. But to be honest, I am not sure if I really want to.

Doctor: I have the impression that you are still divided on the inside. One part very clearly recognizes that you are addicted to alcohol and need help. Another part does not want to quit drinking and is fearful what might happen during a possible treatment. You are faced with a decision in which there are reasons for and against.

Stage 3: Action Phase

This includes emphasizing the freedom of choice, to encourage abstinence and to create a plan for change, together with the patient.

Motivation is not seen as something static, rather as a dynamic, process-like procedure, which requires a specific approach for each phase.

Stage 4: Maintenance Phase

Relapse is more a rule than exception, it is not an addiction-specific phenomenon, but is a part of the 'normal' course of the disease. Outpatient follow-up (self-help groups, counselling, psychotherapy) prevents and can catch incipient relapses effectively. Recidivists avoid self-help groups more often than abstainers, even though the groups are extremely helpful, especially for them.

How Can We Prevent Individual Relapses?

- Early recognition and acceptance of risk situations
- Preparing and practicing possible actions in a risk situation (development of appropriate abstinence thought, planning response options)
- Making lifestyle changes (creating positive dependencies, long-term preventive measures)
- Dealing with the shock of a relapse in case of a slip
- Continuous monitoring

Case Study 'Dialogue after relapse'—relapse management

Patient: I don't know how that could happen. I thought I had everything under control.

Doctor: You are desperate and angry. But the important thing is that you have come here.

Patient: I thought I had it under control.

Doctor: Relapses do occur. This is perfectly normal. The important thing is that we now jointly and constructively deal with the relapse.

Patient: What do we do for him now?

Doctor: My suggestion is that you now go to the hospital immediately for the withdrawal treatment.

Patient: What, to the hospital? Doctor, is this really necessary?

Doctor: Yes. This is now the safest place where you can secure your long-term abstinence.

Pitfalls

The doctor distances himself/herself too much. It is difficult to maintain the balance between therapeutic distance and empathetic closeness. The distancing of the doctor in spite of desires for closeness of the addict leads to the loss of the ability to empathize. The behaviour towards the addict is formalized, the doctor responds mechanically to rule violations, without differentiated assessment of the current situation. There is mistrust and distance between the doctor and the patient.

The doctor has not maintained enough distance. He/she is buddy-buddy with the patient to get closer to him/her. He/she tends to play down and cover up the patient's apparent misconduct, e.g. by issuing certificates of convenience. He/she denies the extent of the addiction, though already several attempts of outpatient treatment have failed and inpatient treatment is urgently needed.

At the first meeting, the patient fools the doctor into believing that he/she was the only one who could help him/her out of this plight. The doctor does not recognize the deception, is committed and takes responsibility for the patient's problems. Sooner or later, his/her idealistic commitment breaks down. He/she retreats disappointedly and angrily: 'Never again I will take care of an alcoholic. They cannot be helped. I'm bitterly disappointed'. The patient is looking for the next saviour.

Through his/her behaviour, the doctor may be counterproductive, disease-prolonging and thus co-dependent if he/she believes that addiction is treatable through medical consultations or on an outpatient basis with medication, without requiring abstinence from the patient.

Cooperation

Usually, an effective addiction treatment can be carried out only in designated outpatient treatment centres and specialized clinics. The withdrawal phase lasts 2–4 weeks, followed by a longer-term psychological detoxification treatment. For logical reasons, this is followed by several month-long outpatient follow-ups in an addiction advice centre and attending a support group.

Internet Addiction

The number of Internet users in clinical practice who fail to make adequate use of the Internet World-Wide Web is increasing (Young 1998). Current national and international studies estimate that 2–7 % of the regular Internet users have problems handling the Internet, from less to more internet-addictive behaviour. The prevalence of Internet addiction is generally higher for adolescents than for adults and higher for men than for women. While addiction in the USA with a 5.7 % prevalence is not significantly different from the European figures, a study from Taiwan identified 17.9 % of adolescents and young adults as people with pathological Internet use.

Professional help is sought very late, mostly following an escalation in the family environment. Despite considerable suffering of patients and their relatives, Internet addiction is not yet recognized as a separate disorder. There are neither consistent diagnostic nor empirically based psychotherapeutic treatment approaches.

Symptoms and Diagnostic Classification

Pathological Internet use is characterized by excessive use of the Internet and loss of control with respect to mostly specific forms of use such as online computer games, chat and messaging, use and/or creation of pornographic Web content. Sufferers report symptoms showing parallels to substance-related addictions such as an intense craving, continuing use despite negative consequences such as declining performance, health problems, intra-family conflicts, withdrawal symptoms when consumption is prevented and the development of tolerance (excessive usage times). Neuroscientific evidence has shown similar cortical processing features like substance-related addictions.

Treatment Goals for Internet Addiction

The main objectives are to reduce the online time to a normal level and the relearning of alternative behaviours. Psychoeducational elements and the communication of functional stress-coping strategies represent a component of treatment.

Cultural Aspects

Asia

A review in 2008 demonstrated that economic and sociocultural factors influenced alcohol consumption greatly in Asia (Chen and Yin 2008). For example, countries influenced more by Buddhism, such as Thailand and Japan, seem to have higher alcohol consumption than those countries mostly influenced by Judaism or Islam. In Taiwan, prevalence rate of alcoholism varied greatly among population of different ethnic backgrounds. The Han Chinese has much lower prevalence rate than the aboriginal people. This difference is related to a genetic factor, namely the aldehyde dehydrogenase deficiency, which is much more common in Han Chinese (Chen et al. 1991).

In Vietnam, alcohol was considered as an essential component in social communication. It has become a Vietnamese cultural trait in wedding, festival, party, etc. Alcohol seems to be good for health, especially when people put some special traditional medications in it. Alcohol was homemade by farmers without any control of quality and consumption. Abuse and dependence rate of alcohol has not been available in Vietnam, but it is estimated that 0.3–3 % of population is dependent.

Internet addiction also constitutes a far-reaching problem. Among Chinese adolescents, the number of those who have a problem with Internet use is on the rise. A nationwide survey (Hui et al. 2011) was conducted in eight Chinese cities involving 17,599 students. Approximately 8 % of all participants reported problematic use of the Internet. Compared with adolescents who use this medium to a normal extent, they often lack physical energy, have physiological dysfunctions and a weakened immune system, suffer from emotional disorders and have difficulty adapting to their social environment. Overall, they are significantly less satisfied with their lives.

Also, in Vietnam, Internet independence is now spreading among young people. Data from the community have not been available. The dependents manifest by spending excess time on Internet, which makes them truant, sleepless, tired, exhausted and violent, when they are impeded.

Africa

Alcohol use in Uganda, like in many other world cultures, is a widely accepted social activity. It is embedded in the local culture and tradition. It is an integral part of the whole village culture and a catalyst in social interactions. Cultural functions such as weddings, births, deaths and funeral rites and circumcision ceremonies cannot be complete without alcohol. Culture is implicated in high level of alcohol consumption in Uganda. For example, in some cultural groups, when a child is given a name, it is also given alcohol to mark the occasion. The fact that alcohol is included in customs signifies the importance of alcohol in people's lives.

Latin America

According to WHO, 8–15 % of the burden of disease in Latin America is attributable to alcohol, as compared to 4 % worldwide (WHO 2002). Brazil, the largest country in South America, provides data indicating that the consumption of alcohol by its population has been growing substantially in the last decade particularly in young people.

The extreme tolerance of the Brazilian society regarding alcohol consumption is considered as intrinsically cultural to Brazil. Examples of this include alcohol behaviour by young males, often considered positively as 'macho behaviour'; the lack of regulations; and the generalised presence of alcoholic beverages in the majority of gatherings and festivals such as carnival, soccer games, parties, funerals and many other events.

In Brazil, the Ministry of Health has recently adopted a multi-professional approach by means of creating specific institutions, which are at the moment mostly located in the bigger cities, named CAPSad—Centro de Atençao Psicossocial Alcool e Drogas (Center for Psychological Care for Alcohol and other Drug Addict). The operational philosophy of these intervention centres is to keep the patient within the family context, and the family also receives psychosocial support. The CAPSad looks after kids, adolescents and adults within group and individual assistance which comprises of social assistance, psychological work, physical exercises, occupational therapies and educational activities. Significant studies to evaluate the CAPESad outcomes are still scarce. Nonetheless, some research findings have indicated that this model is managing to produce positive outcomes.

There are a variety of support programmes in progress to help families of drug addicts, in which the main aims are to reduce anxiety and depression, as well as to improve interpersonal relations. These projects mainly help those family members who face difficulties in coping with stress outcomes of having a drug addict in their homes. It is the case of the PROAD (Programa de Orientaçao e Atendimento a dependentes—Departamento de Psiquiatria—UNIFESP). This program, as well as other similar ones more directly related to the patient, sponsored by university institution, are generally free of charge and mostly run on volunteer or semi-volunteer basis. Studies developed on the outcomes of such interventions have shown significant reduction of depression and anxiety in couples, though not the same positive outcomes were evidenced in cases of single persons. Moreover, this kind of intervention has also been important for a successful outcome for the drug addict patient.

References

Chen CC, Hwu HG, Yeh EK, Morimoto K, Otsuki S. Aldehyde dehydrogenase deficiency, flush patterns and prevalence of alcoholism: an interethnic comparison. Acta Med Okayama. 1991;45(6):409–16.

Chen CC, Yin SJ. Alcohol abuse and related factors in Asia. Int Rev Psychiatry. 2008;20(5):425–33.

Hui C, Ying S, Yuhui W, Jiahu H, Fangbiao T. Problematic Internet use in Chinese adolescents and its relation to psychosomatic symptoms and life satisfaction. BMC Public Health. 2011;11:802.

Miller WR, Rollick S. Motivational interviewing: preparing people to change addictive behavior. New York:Guilford Press; 1991.

Prochaska JO, DiClemente CC. Toward a comprehensive model of change. In: Miller W, Heather N, editors. Addictive behaviour: process of change. New York: Plenum Press; 1986. pp. 3–28.

WHO. World Health Report. Reducing risks, promoting healthy life. 2002. http://www.who.int/whr/2002/en/whr02_en.pdf.

Wittchen HU, Jacobi F, Rehm J, Gustavsson A, Svensson M, Jönsson B, et al. The size and burden of mental disorders and other disorders of the brain in Europe 2010. Eur Neuropsychopharmacol. 2011;21:655–79.

Young KS. Caught in the net. New York: Wiley; 1998.

Part IV
Developing Psychosomatic Medicine in International Settings

Chapter 16
Systems Development of Behavioral Health in Primary Care

Julie Schirmer and Jeffrey F. Markuns

Case Study In 1998, two visiting medical school deans and a health care researcher from Vietnam tour five family medicine training programs in the Philippines and the USA to explore if family medicine training is right for their country. On the last day of this tour, a behavioral health provider and trainer spends the morning with them, giving them a behavioral health overview. Two months later, she makes the first of what turns out to be annual or biannual trips to Asia over a 15-year period to assist with training and systems development. Over a 15-year period, this provider and team have worked with schools of medicine, social work, and different levels of the health care and government to strategize how to best integrate behavioral health first into family medicine training and clinical care and second into social work training and service. This team's work in Vietnam, Laos, and Cambodia continues to involve (1) training medical providers and the rest of the primary health care team, (2) advocacy to policy makers and administrators, (3) establishing primary care clinics affiliated with the training programs, and (4) encouraging campaigns to reduce stigma.

J. Schirmer (✉)
Family Medicine Department Maine Medical Center,
Family Medicine Center, 272 Congress Street,
Portland, ME 04101, USA
e-mail: jschirme4@gmail.com

J. F. Markuns
Department of Family Medicine, Boston University,
771 Albany Street Dowling 5,
South Boston, MA 02118. USA
e-mail: jeffrey.markuns@bmc.org

K. Fritzsche et al. (eds.), *Psychosomatic Medicine,* DOI 10.1007/978-1-4614-1022-5_16,

Table 16.1 The core principles of behavioral medicine health educators in primary care

Those who apply these principles
1. Use biopsychosocial- and relationship-centered approaches to care
2. Promote patient self-efficacy and behavior change as primary factors in health promotion, disease prevention, and chronic disease management
3. Integrate psychological and behavioral knowledge into the care of physical symptoms and diseases
4. Promote the integration of sociocultural factors within the organization and delivery of health care services
5. Practice a developmental and life-cycle perspective with learners and clients; and
6. Encourage and support provider self-awareness, empathy, and well-being. (Society of Teachers of Family Medicine 2009)

Definition

Behavioral health is a term that has been in the literature since the late 1970s. It is defined as "the reciprocal relationship between human behavior and the well-being of the body, mind, and spirit, whether considered individually or as an integrated whole" (Patient Centered Primary Care Collaborative 2012). It includes mental health care, substance abuse care, health behavior change, and attention to family and other psychosocial issues. Behavioral health has a broad focus that includes prevention, diagnosis, treatment, and rehabilitation. It encompasses the terms *behavioral medicine*, which is the interdisciplinary field of behavioral health (Society of Teachers of Family Medicine 2012) and behavioral science, which provides the evidence to support behavioral health practices. These terms have been used interchangeably over the years. We will use the term behavioral health throughout this chapter, considering it the more inclusive term. Behavioral health providers can include primary care physicians, assistant physicians, psychiatrists, nurse practitioners, nurses, social workers, psychologists, counselors, midwives, and community health workers. Each discipline plays a different role and has different levels of training and responsibility for addressing the behavioral health needs of an office practice or a community. The core principles of behavioral medicine health educators in primary care are listed in Table 16.1.

Training resources include a Behavioral Science Basics Wiki, which provides free, up-to-date resources for persons who train primary medical providers in behavioral health care (Family Medicine Digital Resource Library 2012). The University of Massachusetts and others provide a 6 month, 6 day online training course for behavioral health providers in primary care (Certificate Program in Primary Behavioral Health 2012).

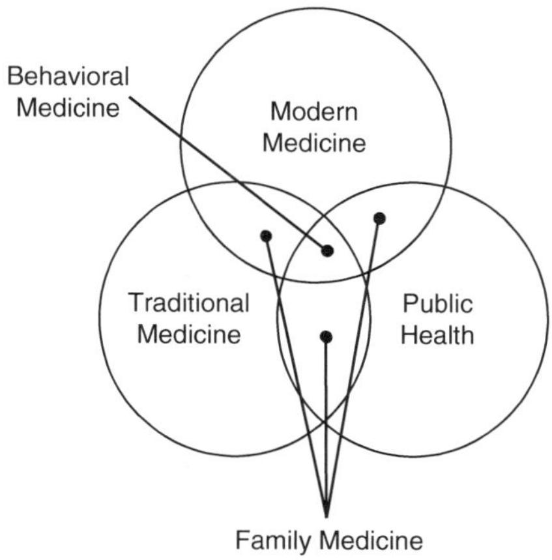

Fig. 16.1 The three components of the biopsychosocial–spiritual model

Theory

Biopsychosocial–Spiritual Theory (See Also Chap. 1 "What is Psychosomatic Medicine?")

The biopsychosocial–spiritual model provides the conceptual framework for the practice of behavioral health. Many add the spiritual component to George Engle's biopsychosocial model, emphasizing the importance of spirituality in one's perception of health, illness, and death. The biopsychosocial–spiritual model is at the intersection of modern medicine, traditional medicine, and public health (Fig. 16.1). Modern medicine involves the biomedical causes, treatment, rehabilitation, and management of diseases, including mental illness and substance abuse issues. Traditional medicine honors the familial, cultural, and spiritual perspectives of the patient, involves the impact of a community or group on the patient, and acknowledges and interprets the impact of stress on the body. Public health involves the study of social, economic, and environmental factors that impact the health of a community. The public health world includes the social determinants of health, which both the individual patient and health care provider predominantly have very little control over.

Medical Anthropology Theory

Medical anthropology and medical sociology are fields of study looking at cultural issues and how they relate to health and health care (Scrimshaw 2001). This approach involves:

- Learning about common beliefs and practices

- Understanding how the local culture's family structures, values, and everyday activities shape systems of care or how different health or mental health interventions might work in the local context
- Being aware of other professionals', lay practitioners', and, most importantly, patients' perceptions of healthcare and healing

Organization Theory

The Three World View of Systems Change recommends that every action designed to produce a change in an organization or system must satisfy the demands of the clinical, operational, and financial worlds (Peek 2008). In health care, including behavioral health, *the clinical world* involves how patients are assessed, diagnosed, and treated. *The operational world* involves how patients move through the health care and behavioral health care systems, and the processes these systems use to function in a productive way. *The financial world* involves how the care is financed, the costs of providing the service, and the net gains and losses. The practice section below suggests ways to address these worlds when developing behavioral health care training and care in low-to-moderate income countries.

Practice

The Example: Vietnam

After the team's initial 5-year consultation, the Vietnam Ministry of Health acknowledged the need for family medicine and declared that all medical schools need to develop training programs in family medicine. Although, training programs in the medical schools and a national family medicine curriculum was approved, the government had not approved full funding of these training programs. With the help of several international health care funders, the Ministries of Health and Education, five medical schools, and select provincial and district health systems, the consultants continued to work on developing family medicine training and systems over the following decade.

Support for behavioral health could come from psychiatrists at the medical schools and the traditional medical physicians. There were three psychiatry training programs in the major cities of Hanoi, Hue, and Ho Chi Minh City and no professional counseling training programs (Schirmer et al. 2004).

The Example: Laos

Although they are neighbors, the Laos medical and behavioral systems looked and operated very differently. Starting in 2002, US consultants began visiting Laos, to meet with government and medical school leaders to explore family medicine training and resource development. The process of how things get done and medical and psychosocial needs as defined by the government looked very different between Laos and Vietnam. Compared with Vietnam, Laos is extremely low resourced, especially in the area of human resources for health. Laos had two psychiatrists, one masters level social work school, and one medical school, all of which were in Vientiane, the capital of Laos. Social work training focused on women and children.

Laos and Vietnam share a border, but their economies were very different. The per capita income in Vietnam was more than US$ 200/year higher than in Laos, allowing more total money to be dedicated to health and mental health care education and training.

Tensions

A country's economic, political, and health care structures tremendously influence the country's readiness to focus efforts on behavioral and mental health care. The national health care infrastructure and national priorities—including both the political and economic—dictate the degree of development of the primary care and behavioral health care systems.

When working in countries different from one's own, it is important to know who else is doing behavioral health development work in the country. The in-country behavioral health champions may not necessarily inform you of the work of other consultants. It is important to ask in-country champions directly about these matters and seek out these other consultants in order to enhance each other's efforts and not work at cross-purposes. Developing countries typically are operating with both, limited financial and human resources. Well-intentioned but duplicative, competing, or uncoordinated programs can quickly overtax a nation's available committed resources for the task. Key tensions which influence the development of mental and behavioral health systems are summarized in Table 16.2.

Opportunities

The WHO and the UK have developed key strategies for mental health development (Garrison 2012) These strategies, along with the authors' recommendations, are incorporated into the Tables 16.3–16.5, which are organized according to the financial, clinical, and operational domains of the Three World View of Systems Change.

A consensus statement of national and international US experts delineating the principles for successful behavioral health integration into primary care has been created by a leading panel of national and international US experts. These principles affirm the strategies outlined above and are listed in Table 16.6.

Table 16.2 Key tensions which influence the development of mental and behavioral health systems

Tension between horizontally integrating behavioral health into the primary care system versus developing vertical-based specialty behavioral health systems. Where resources are few, behavioral health specialists may work more effectively as consultants, supervisors, and trainers to primary care providers
Tension of training professionals (psychiatrists, family physicians, professional nurses, midwives, or social workers) versus training nonspecialist behavioral health providers (communal health workers, spiritual advisors, clergy, or community leaders). The evidence has illustrated that trained nonspecialists can provide effective mental health with sustainable results (Patel 2003; Bolton 2003)
Tensions between the different ministries within a country
Tension between different cultural perspectives about the cause and treatment of mental health
Tension between the medical model of behavioral health that involves diagnosis and treatment versus the "personal fault" model given to persons with these disorders
Tension between consultants focused on specific health care clinic development (i.e., those who go to create and set up health, mental health, and social service clinics in low-resourced areas) versus consultants focused on training and larger system development (i.e., those who primarily develop system-based infrastructure to advance a nation's overall education and health care system)

Table 16.3 Financial strategies for country-wide mental health development

Financial domain
Financial and human resources are needed (WHO/Wonca 2008)
Policy and plans need to incorporate primary care for mental health (WHO/Wonca 2008), eventually on a national scale. This involves legislating and funding curricula, training centers, job codes for new specialties, and system changes
National policy must allow for flexibility, based on community need (New Ways of Working 2011)
Relationship development is needed with persons in pertinent government and nongovernment agencies affiliated with health, education, finance, labor, and social services

Table 16.4 Clinical strategies for country-wide mental health development

Clinical domain
Epidemiological studies must identify the prevalence and needs in the country so that politicians and leaders can see the significance and not discount mental health and behavioral health problems
Adequate training of teachers and practitioners is essential (WHO/Wonca 2008) and must include multiple providers such as psychiatrists, family physicians, social workers, and nurses
Primary care tasks on behavioral and mental health must be focused, limited, and doable (WHO/Wonca 2008)
Primary care providers must have access to psychiatric and behavioral specialty supervision and support for sustainability purposes (WHO/Wonca 2008)
Patients must have access to essential psychotropic medications (WHO/Wonca 2008)
Quality improvement studies are needed to identify what is feasible and effective, and to improve care and policy

Cultural Aspects

The Three World View described in this chapter must take into account the cultural differences and similarities between consultants and advisees. Strategies to address culture are listed in Table 16.7.

Table 16.5 Operational strategies for country-wide mental health development

Operational domain
A behavioral health service coordinator is needed (WHO/Wonca 2008)
Protocols linking specialty mental health professionals and primary care providers must be developed
Referral pathways are needed for patients with severe and chronic mental illness (New Ways of Working 2011)
Patients and caregivers must be involved in the process of developing and maintaining mental health and behavioral health-care services (Garrison 2012)
Integration must be seen as an on-going process, not an event (WHO/Wonca 2008)
Partnering with community agencies, nongovernment agencies, village health workers, and volunteers is required (WHO/Wonca 2008)
Advocacy and social marketing will educate communities, reduce stigma, and increase access to treatment (Garrison 2012)

Table 16.6 Principles for successful behavioral health integration into primary care

Agreement on clear and consistent language across disciplines, particularly on the terms behavioral health, mental health, and behavioral change
Understanding of the central role of the patient and family in articulating needs and developing a plan of care
Defining the different roles and skill sets required for physicians, behavioral health clinicians, and other members of the health-care team to provide whole-person care
Interdisciplinary training offered to practicing clinicians and other team members, faculty fellows, residents, and students for the roles that behavioral health clinicians, primary care clinicians, and other team members will assume when integrated into a primary care system
Research to better define the optimal provision of behavioral health integration, with attention to patient, practice, training, and financing issues
Recognition of local adaptations of integrated, whole-person care so as to include all persons and to take advantage of the differing requirements and resources of different communities across a region or country
Assurance that behavioral health services are appropriately financed

Table 16.7 Strategies to address culture

Recruit the insider and outsider perspective. The US consultants strategically recruited Vietnamese consulting teachers who were physicians and insiders to the medical culture and others who were well-respected "outsiders" to the Vietnamese medical system
Recognize and address stigma at all levels. There are many successful strategies that spell out best practice in this area that can positively affect patients, improve primary care providers' knowledge, skills, and confidence in addressing these issues (Garrison 2012)

Conclusion

Behavioral health systems are best developed alongside primary care systems development in low and moderate income countries. Many lessons are to be learned from countries where this has not been the case and the care is fragmented. Using Vietnam and Laos examples, key theories, principles and strategies are outlined to assist in integrating behavioral health into a nation's health care system.

References

Bolton P, Bass J, Neugebauer R, Verdeli H, Clougherty KF, Wickmaratne P, et al. Group interpersonal psychotherapy for depression in rural Uganda: a randomized controlled trial. JAMA. 2003; 289(23):3117–24.

Certificate Program for Primary Behavioral Health. Center for integrated primary care. University of Massachusetts Medical School. 2012. http://www.umassmed.edu/cipc/pcbhoverview.aspx?linkidentifier=id&itemid=144778. Accessed: 23 July 2012.

Garrison P, Ivbijaro G, Ennum Y, Maguire D, Schirmer JM, Franciosi P. Advocacy and overcoming stigma in primary care mental health. In: Ivbijaro G, editor. Companion to primary care mental health. Oxford: Radcliffe Publishers; 2012.

New Ways of Working. New ways of working for primary care in mental health. 2011. http://www.newwaysofworking.org.uk/content/view/56/467/. Accessed: 2 Nov. 2011.

Patel V. Where there is no psychiatrist: a mental health manual. London: Gaskell; 2003.

Patient Centered Primary Care Collaborative. Behavioral health defined. 2012. http://www.pcpcc.net/behavioral-health.html. Accessed: 12 June 2012.

Peek CJ. Planning care in the clinical, operational, and financial worlds. In: Kessler R, Stafford D, editors. Collaborative medicine case studies: evidence in practice. New York: Springer; 2008.

Schirmer JM and Ninh HL. The Vietnam Family Medicine Development Project: A Cross Cultural Collaboration. Families, Systems and Health. 2012. 20: 303–310.

Schirmer JM, Cartwright C, Montegut AJ, Dreher GK, Stovall J. A collaborative needs assessment and work plan in behavioral medicine curriculum development in Vietnam. Fam Syst Health. 2004;22(4):410–8.

Schirmer JM. Society of teachers of family medicine resource library, society of teachers of family medicine. 2012. http://www.fmdrl.org/group/index.cfm?event=c.showWikiHome&wikiId=85. Accessed: 12 June 2012.

Scrimshaw C. Culture, behaviour, and health. In: Merson MH, Black RE, Mills AJ, editors. International public health: diseases, programs, systems, and policies. Gaithersburg: Aspen Publishers; 2001.

Schirmer JM and Ninh LH. Behavioral medicine: principles and practices. In: Schirmer, JM and Montegut AM, editors. Behavioral Medicine in Primary Care: A Global Perspective, Oxford: Radcliffe Publishers; 2009.

Society of Teachers of Family Medicine Resource Library, Behavioral Science Basics Wiki. http://www.fmdrl.org/group/index.cfm?event=c.showWikiHome&wikiId=85 Accessed June 12, 2012.

World Health Organization (WHO) and the World Organization of Family Doctors (Wonca). Integrating mental health into primary care: a global perspective. Geneva: WHO; 2008.

Chapter 17
The Development of Psychosomatic Medicine in China, Vietnam, and Laos—The ASIA-LINK Program

Kurt Fritzsche, Michael Wirsching, Xudong Zhao, Jing Wei, Lan Zhang, Kim Viet Nguyen and Van Tuan Nguyen

Background

In different ways, China, Vietnam, and Laos have undergone major social, economic, and cultural changes. Traditional values are being questioned or are disappearing, and new social values and structures have not yet been established. Despite significant

K. Fritzsche (✉) · M. Wirsching
Department of Psychosomatic Medicine and Psychotherapy,
University Medical Center, Hauptstr. 8, 79104 Freiburg, Germany
e-mail: kurt.fritzsche@uniklinik-freiburg.de

M. Wirsching
e-mail: michael.wirsching@uniklinik-freiburg.de

X. Zhao
Department of Psychosomatic Medicine,
Shanghai East Hospital Affiliated to Tongji University, 150 Jimo Road,
Pudong New Area, 200120 Shanghai, China
e-mail: zhaoxd@tongji.edu.cn

J. Wei
Department of Psychological Medicine, Peking Union Medical College Hospital,
1 Shuaifuyuan, Dongcheng District, 100730 Beijing, China
e-mail: weijing@pumch.cn

L. Zhang
Department of Psychiatry, West China Hospital, No. 37 Guoxue Lane,
Chengdu, 610041 Sichuan, P.R. China
e-mail: lanzhang3@gmail.com

K. V. Nguyen · V. T. Nguyen
Department of Psychiatry, Hanoi Medical University,
No. 1, Ton That Tung Street, Dong Da District, Hanoi, Vietnam
e-mail: drnkimviet@yahoo.com

National Institute of Mental Health, Bach Mai Hospital,
No. 78, Giai Phong Road, Dong Da District, Hanoi, Vietnam

V. T. Nguyen
e-mail: nvtuannimhvn@hmu.edu.vn

K. Fritzsche et al. (eds.), *Psychosomatic Medicine,* DOI 10.1007/978-1-4614-1022-5_17,

increases in the wealth of the population, particularly in the cities, there have been simultaneous increases in uncertainty and in stressful living situations for a large majority of the population. As a result of these social upheavals, psychological and psychosomatic disorders and problems are on the rise (World Health Organization (WHO). The World Health report 2001; Patel and Kleinman 2003; Lopez et al. 2006; Prince et al. 2007; Saxena et al. 2007).

In Southeast Asia, 11 % of disability-adjusted life years and 27 % of years lived with disabilities are the results of neuropsychiatric disease (Lopez et al. 2006). Depression is the largest contributor to this disease burden (World Health Report 2001). The majority of the patients, who suffer from common mental disorders (CMDs), such as depressive and anxiety disorders, seek help in primary care. The point prevalence of CMDs in South Asian primary care practices varies between 20 and 45 %. A review of eight epidemiological studies of CMDs in South Asia showed that their point prevalence in primary care was 26.3 % (95 % CI, 25.3–27.4 %). Less than one-third of clinically significant CMDs are recognized (Ustun and Von Korff 1995; Xiao et al. 1997; Patel 1999; Yu et al. 2004). The resulting chronicity causes severe burdens on the affected families and on the health system.

In contrast, East Asia, particularly China, has a health system that is based on high-tech Western medicine. But there are only about 20,000 registered psychiatrists in China. Moreover, most of them used to focus on psychosis diagnosis and treatment.

Basic care is lacking for common mental and psychosomatic disorders and problems, and this care is not adequately addressed by traditional medicine. In the current medical education systems in China and Vietnam, psychosomatic or psychological content is only marginally taught (Tao 1994; Schirmer and Ninh 2002; Montegut et al. 2004; Liu 2005; Schirmer et al. 2005). More psychiatric education is available; however, it is taught mostly, if not always, in a biological manner, and there is a strong emphasis on psychotropic drugs and custodial care. Psychiatric resources are also lacking, which often allows the treatment of only severe cases, such as psychosis. In Vietnam, there is one psychiatrist for every 300,000 inhabitants. Only half of the eight medical schools have first-degree specialty training programs in psychiatry. Psychologists administer psychological tests and sometimes perform consultations, primarily in schools and industry (Schirmer and Ninh 2002; Montegut et al. 2004; Schirmer et al. 2005). Furthermore, education about consultation-liaison psychiatry and psychosomatics in daily clinical practice is nonexistent (Zhao et al. 1998; Yu et al. 2004). The situation in Laos is even worse: For the entire country, there are only two trained psychiatrists in the capital, Vientiane.

It is apparent that the current medical education systems in China, Vietnam, and Laos need support in different ways to develop efficient educational institutions and care structures.

From 2005 to 2008, a European–Asian cooperative project funded by the European Union was coordinated by Freiburg University (Department of Psychosomatic Medicine and Psychotherapy). The objective of the project was to support the development of Psychosomatic Medicine in China (Tongji University), Vietnam (Universities of Ho Chi Minh City and Hue), and Laos (University of Vientiane). In this project, a basic psychosomatic care curriculum for postgraduate medical doctors was applied.

The Project

During the first year, a team of prospective teachers was recruited for each center. The didactic elements of the new curriculum were taught to the future teachers. This was a mutual process that involved the German team teaching the teachers and adapting, modifying, and redesigning the lessons within the context of the partners. Teaching the teachers served as an experimental curriculum while supporting the future independence of the partners from the assistance of the European experts. The experimental lessons followed the contents of the intended curriculum. Teaching the teachers, therefore, focused on three target areas:

- Teaching both the content of the biopsychosocial approach in medicine and the topics included in the planned curriculum
- Teaching didactic methods, strategies, and skills for managing and teaching the lessons; and
- Adapting the teaching methods to specific contexts.

At the end of this activity, the future teachers were able to manage the pilot curriculum with the assistance of their European partners during the second year.

During the third year, the Asian partners were encouraged to organize and implement the new curriculum on their own. The results of the evaluations and the partners' accumulated competence helped to fit the curriculum elements to the needs of the partners. The European staff provided supervision but limited their participation in teaching the curriculum (except for roles as guest lecturers on special topics). Supervisors supported the teachers' needs in managing the courses and becoming competent trainers of biopsychosocial skills.

More information and an overview of the 3-year program, including the experimental and supervision phases, can be found in a previously published report (Fritzsche et al. 2008).

Results

Regional training centers were formed In China (Shanghai), Vietnam (Ho Chi Minh City and Hue), and Laos (Vientiane). A total of 200 physicians completed the training, and 30 physicians acquired the status of future teacher. The acceptance of the training was high, and feelings of competence increased during the courses. The interactive training methods were greatly appreciated, with the skills training and self-experience ranked as the most important topics. Adaptations to the cultural background of the participants were necessary for the topics of "breaking bad news," the handling of negative emotions, discontinuities in participation, the hierarchical doctor–patient relationship, culture-specific syndromes, and language barriers. In addition to practical skills for daily clinical practice, the participants wanted to learn more about didactic teaching methods. Half a year after the completion of the training program, the participants stated that the program had a great impact on their daily medical practice.

Misunderstandings and Cultural Adaptions

The results in this section are derived from the interviews with the future teachers and from debriefings of the course teachers.

Handling of Negative Emotions

Chinese culture emphasizes the inhibition of strong emotional expression (Li 1985; Ots 1990; Lee 1997). Young children are sometimes scolded by their mothers for aggressive behavior (Bond and Hwang 1986). In our communication skills training, we introduced elements of "active listening" (Rogers 1942, 1997), which include "mirroring emotions," naming perceived feelings, and showing these emotions through nonverbal displays of anger or sadness, for example. Because of their cultural background, this communication behavior was met with resistance by the participants. The essentially empathic nature of the Rogers approach was not questioned, nor was the usefulness of empathic support during difficult emotional situations, e.g., during discussions of a life-threatening disease or critical life events. However, the expression of personal concerns or feelings in difficult doctor–patient relationships was rejected, e.g., if the patient were upset and angry because he/she experienced a prolonged wait. In this case, a statement such as "I can understand that you are very angry" or "If I were you, I would be upset, too" would be considered an admission of guilt by the doctor. Such an admission would be associated with a loss of authority over the patient and could cause the patient to change doctors.

Balint Groups, Sculpture Work, and Reflecting Teams (see also Chap. 8 "Balint Group")

It is foreign to some Asian cultures to discuss negative feelings outside the family (Lee 1997). During the first Balint group sessions, these traditions were repeatedly confirmed by the future trainers. Our experience with classical Balint work appeared to confirm that the participants felt overwhelmed by the instruction to express their thoughts, feelings, and fantasies freely. Subsequently, we modified the classical Balint work by the introduction of sculpture. This modification completely changed the results: the participants became absorbed in their roles; they spoke of their fears, their anger, and their sadness; and they identified with the people they represented. In this way, sculpture facilitated vivacity and improved doctor–patient dynamics. The doctor–patient relationship was part of the system and was improved by a change in the position of the doctor, which resulted in decreased symptoms and improved well-being on the part of the patients.

Family Norms and "Breaking Bad News" (see also Chap. 12 "Psycho-Oncology")

For the physicians in the three countries involved in the program, disclosing diagnoses and prognoses to patients is extremely challenging. Most Asian families ask doctors not to reveal the diagnoses and prognoses of family members (Hu et al. 2002). One reason for this request might be families' fear that a loved one suffering from cancer will despair and become hopeless upon learning of their diagnoses (Tse et al. 2003). The methods of delivering bad news in oncology are influenced by cultural diversity (Ong et al. 2002). In Western countries, oncologists usually inform cancer patients of their diagnoses (Grassi et al. 2000).

When patients follow the principle of autonomy and families follow the principle of beneficence in disclosing information about cancer, physicians find themselves in a dilemma (Wang et al. 2004). Doctors need support in solving this dilemma and determining what to tell cancer patients. In our communication skills training, we addressed this dilemma and tried to find solutions for it in specific cases. We must find a balance between disclosing information about cancer and the needs of patients and families. We took seriously physicians' concerns about disclosing information about cancer diagnoses, and we carefully sought ways to solve the conflict between the patient's right to be informed and the traditional norms of the Asian family without harming the patient. In Asian cultures, the principles of family decision-making and family involvement in decision-making are paramount and constitute an integral part of the self-concept of the individual (Fan 1997). This cultural characteristic should be appropriately recognized and acknowledged.

Future training sessions will continue to address this issue, in an attempt to find a family-centered approach (Back and Huak 2005) of breaking bad news to the patient and his/her family.

Doctor–Patient Relationship

The doctor–patient relationship in all three Asian countries can be described as patriarchal and is characterized by a doctor-centered mode of communication. Patients expect the doctor to be the expert and to tell them what to do. Patient-centered interviewing is unusual in Asia.

The patients in the live patient interviews and the participating physicians appreciated the empathic, respectful, patient-centered interview style. However, the German teachers were also considered "famous professors from abroad," from whom cures for their ailments were expected. Due to the traditional norms, a cooperative doctor–patient relationship with a patient-centered interview style might not be immediately implemented in everyday life. Elements of patient-centered communication skills such as short breaks, summarizing, and questions regarding subjective health have proven to be highly teachable and learnable as a first entry into different attitudes and a better design of the doctor–patient relationship.

High Performance Pressure

In most general outpatient clinics and in outpatient psychiatric and Psychosomatic Medicine clinics, 30–60 patients are seen by one doctor in a single morning; in large hospitals in China, a total of up to 10,000 patients per day are seen. Usually, the doctor has only 2–3 min for each patient. In specialty outpatient clinics, which are usually operated by experienced specialists and are rather expensive, the doctors might have 10–15 min. This high performance pressure raises doubts about whether the diagnostic and therapeutic skills learned in the training sessions can be applied in everyday practice. We recommended that the participants initially gather psychosocial histories from selected patients and provide supportive care only when there is a sufficient time frame of 10–15 min.

Impacts on the Health Care System

Primary care is part of community hospital health center-based services (Schirmer et al. 2005). In outpatient clinics, there is little room for individual, personal doctor–patient relationships, which frequently form the basis of successful treatment. Somatizing patients in China often complain about a lack of understanding of their complaints by their doctors and about a lack of treatment success (Meng et al. 1999). Conversely, a WHO study of mental disorders in primary care showed that patients with continuous doctor–patient relationships presented with somatic symptoms as frequently as those who did not experience such relationships (Ustun and Von Korff 1995; Simon et al. 1999). Continuous doctor–patient contact and good doctor–patient relationships should be implemented, comparable to the role of the general practitioner in primary care services in Europe and other Anglo-American areas.

In future courses, a more detailed medical history of subjective illness conceptions and expectations would certainly expand our range of knowledge. Future training programs should also include rural areas. In the future, these cultural blind spots can be better addressed through our new insight about these potential misunderstandings and close corporation with our partners (Like 1996; Haq et al. 2000; Galanti 2008; Ring et al. 2008, Schirmer and Montegut 2009; Mostow et al. 2010).

Current and Future Projects

In China and Vietnam, advanced training in Psychosomatic Medicine and psychotherapy has begun. Tongji University in Shanghai, together with the medical faculty of Freiburg, Germany, launched a Master's degree in Psychosomatic Medicine and Psychotherapy in September 2011. In Vietnam, a 4-year program began in November 2011 with three objectives: (1) the introduction and implementation of a three level, modular curriculum on Psychosomatic Medicine and psychotherapy for medical students and doctors; (2) the establishment of this curriculum as a regular part of the national curriculum of medical education on Psychosomatic Medicine and psychotherapy; and (3) the development of international European–Asian networks and the enhancement of intercultural communication.

The ASIA-LINK curriculum has also promoted the development of joint research projects and the exchange of doctors and medical students between Germany and China and Vietnam. Through contact with the Cancer Hospital in Beijing, a training program for Chinese oncologists, "Breaking Bad News," has been developed and scientifically evaluated (Wünsch et al. 2013). The German Robert Bosch Foundation, the German Research Council and the Sino-German Center for Research Promotion in Beijing have supported research projects on illness perception, illness behavior, doctor–patient relationships and the treatment outcomes of patients with medically unexplained physical symptoms (somatoform disorders) in China.

The Chinese government has required setting up Psychosomatic Medicine departments or psychological departments in the tertiary hospitals which represent high service quality hospitals in China. Consequently, it means more well-trained Psychosomatic Medicine doctors are urgently needed. On October 26, 2012 the National People's Congress adopted the first national mental health law of the People's Republic of China. It contains important implications for the integration of mental health in primary care (Mental Health Law of the People's Republic of China 2012).

Under the administration of Professor Zhang Lan a work team of psychiatrists and nurses has been formed in Chengdu pursuing two aims:

1. The scientific explorations of prevalence of psychosocial and psychosomatic problems and disorders in the general hospital and the need of patients and doctors to treat them.
2. Implementation of training programs in Psychosomatic Basic Care for medical doctors and nurses in the general hospitals in Chengdu.

Nurses and medical doctors are counseling and supporting patients with psychosocial problems. If it concerns serious mental disorders they turn to the psychiatric consultation liaison service.

Finally, the experiences with Balint groups in our program led to the establishment of a Chinese Balint society. The first conference, which included international participation, occurred in May 2011. The participants expressed a desire to establish Balint groups at their own hospitals, which has led to a plan to offer a Balint group leader seminar at the next international conference, in June 2012 and 2013.

Conclusions

This project had a significant impact on all of the participants. The course evaluation demonstrated that the medical doctors enrolled in the courses received highly qualified and effective training and demonstrated the participants' progress in both professional competence and self-development. These physicians are now connected by international collaboration and intercultural cooperation. The establishment of national and international networks has been facilitated. The future teachers learned practical clinical skills, didactic, and management skills in applying the training curriculum. They have taken over key responsibilities in continuing and consolidating the future training and education of medical doctors in their countries. The partner university hospitals, as institutional stakeholders, have shown interest in the project and have granted support for further development in this field. The European partners gained valuable experience and competence in international projects and in the successful conduct of intercultural communication. As a result of the exchanges of ideas and practical experience between the Western and Asian medical doctors and patients, new elements can be added to Western treatment theories in Germany, China, Vietnam, and Laos that will help to create promising new research fields. Finally, patients will benefit from an improved mental health care system.

References

Back MF, Huak CY. Family centred decision making and non-disclosure of diagnosis in a South East Asian oncology practice. Psychooncology. 2005;14:1052–9.

Bond MH, Hwang KK. The social psychology of the Chinese people. In: Bond MH, editor. The psychology of the Chinese people. Hong Kong:Oxford University Press; 1986.

Fan R. Self-determination vs. family-determination: two incommensurable principles of autonomy: a report from East Asia. Bioethics. 1997;11:309–22.

Fritzsche K, Scheib P, Wirsching M, Schüßler G, Wu W, Cat NH, et al. Improving the psychosomatic competence of medical doctors in China, Vietnam and Laos—the ASIA-LINK Program. Int J Psychiat Med. 2008;38:1–11.

Galanti GA. Caring for patients from different cultures. Philadelphia: University of Pennsylvania Press; 2008.

Grassi L, Giraldi T, Messina EG, Magnani K, Valle E, Cartei G. Physicians' attitudes to and problems with truth-telling to cancer patients. Support Care Cancer. 2000;8:40–5.

Haq C, Rothenberg D, Gierde C, Bobula J, Wilson C, Bickley L, et al. New world views: preparing physicians in training for global health work. Fam Med. 2000;32:566–72.

Hu WY, Chiu TY, Chuang RB, Chen CY. Solving family-related barriers to truthfulness in cases of terminal cancer in Taiwan. A professional perspective. Cancer Nurs. 2002;25:486–92.

Lee E. Working with Asian-Americans. New York:Guilford Press; 1997.

Li TY. Mental disorders and psychiatry in Chinese culture. In: Tseng WS, Wu DYH, editors. Chinese culture and mental health. Orlando:Academic Press; 1985.

Like RC. Recommended core curriculum guidelines on culturally sensitive and competent health care. Fam Med. 1996;27:291–7.

Liu X. The consideration about the present investigation of medical psychological knowledge of general practitioners and the training strategy. Chinese General Practice. 2005;8(Suppl 17):1397–8. (in Chinese).

Lopez A, Mathers C, Ezzati M, Jamison D, Murray C. Global burden of disease and risk factors. Washington:Oxford University Press and the World Bank; 2006.

Meng F, Cui Y, Shen Y. Perliminary investigation on clinical features of somatoform disorders in general hospital. Chinese Ment Health J. 1999;13:67–9.

Mental Health Law of the People's Republic of China. (English translation with annotations) (Trans. Chen HH, Phillips MR, Chen H, Chen QQ, Chen XD, Fralick D, et al.). Shanghai Archives of Psychiatry. Advance online publication 2012. doi:10.3969/j.issn.1002-0829.2012.06.001.

Montegut AJ, Cartwright C, Schirmer JM, Cummings S. An international consultation: the development of family medicine education in Vietnam. Fam Med. 2004;35:352–60.

Mostow C, Crosson J, Gordon S, Chapman S, Gonzalez P, Hardt E, et al. Treating and precepting with RESPECT: a relational model addressing race, ethnicity, and culture in medical training. J Gen Intern Med. 2010;25:146–54.

Ong KJ. Back MF, Lu JJ, Shakespeare TS, Wynne CJ. Cultural attitudes to cancer management in traditional South-East-Asian patients. Australas Radiol. 2002;46:370–4.

Ots TH. The angy Liver, the anxious heart, and the melancholy spleen. Cult Med Psychiat. 1990;14:21–58.

Patel V. The epidemiology of common mental disorders in South Asia. NIMHANS Jnl. 1999;17:307–27.

Patel V, Kleinman A. Poverty and common mental disorders in developing countries. Bull World Health Organ. 2003;8:609–15.

Prince M, Patel V, Saxena S, Maj M, Maselko J, Phillips M, et al. No health without mental health. The Lancet. 2007;370:859–77.

Ring JM, Nyquist JG, Mitchell S. Curriculum for culturally responsive health care: a step-by-step guide to cultural competence training. Oxford: Radcliffe Publishers; 2008.

Rogers CR. Counseling and psychotherapy. Boston; 1942.

Rogers CR. an unappreciated way of being. Couns Psychol. 1997;5:2–10.

Saxena S, Thornicroft G, Knapp M, Whiteford H. Resources for mental health: scarcity, inequity and inefficiency. The Lancet. 2007;370:878–89.

Schirmer J, Ninh LH. The Vietnam family medicine development project: a cross-cultural collaboration. Fam Syst Health. 2002;20:303–10.

Schirmer JM, Cartwright C, Montegut AJ, Dreher GK, Stovall J. A collaborative needs assessment and work plan in behavioural medicine curriculum development in Vietnam. Fam Syst Health. 2005;22:410–8.

Schirmer J, Montegut A. Behavioral medicine in primary care: a global perspective. Oxford: Radcliffe Publishers; 2009.

Simon GE, von Korff M, Piccinelli M, Fullerton C, Ormel J. An international study of the relation between somatic symptoms and depression. N Engl J Med. 1999;341:1329–35.

Tao Y. The necessary of medical psychology education in traditional Chinese medical college. Traditional Chinese Medicine Education. 1994;3:24. (in Chinese).

Tse CY, Chong A, Fok SY. Breaking bad news: a Chinese perspective. Palliat Med. 2003;17:339–43.

Ustun TB, Von Korff M. Primary mental health services: access and provision of care. In: Ustun TB, Sartorius N, editors. Mental illness in general health care: an international study. Chichester: Wiley; 1995.

Wang SY, Chen CH, Chen YS, Huang HL. The attitude toward truth telling of cancer in Taiwan. J Psychosom Res. 2004;57:53–8.

WHO. The World Health Report: mental health: new understanding, new hope. http://www.who.int/whr2001/en.

Wünsch A, Tang L, Goelz T, Zhang Y, Stubenrauch S, Song L, et al. Breaking bad news in China-the dilemma of patients' rights to be informed and traditional norms. A first communication skills training for Chinese oncologists and caretakers. Psychooncology. 2013;22(5):1192–5. doi: 10.1002/pon.3112.

Xiao SF, Yan HQ, Lu YF, Bi H, Pu JY, Xiao ZPI. World Health Organization collaborative study on psychological disorders in primary health care: the results from Shanghai. Chin J Psychiatry. 1997:30(Suppl 2):90–4.

Yu DH, Wu WY, Zhang MY. Current situation of mental health service in general hospitals in Shanghai. Chin J Psychiatry. 2004;37:176–8.

Zhao XD, Xu XF, Bai Y, Jiang HZ. The retrospective study of psychiatric consultation in general hospital. Chin J Psychiatry. 1998;31(Suppl 4):231–3.

Chapter 18
Psychosomatic Medicine and Its Implementation in the Latin America Region

Sonia Diaz Monsalve

The psychosomatic concept in the Latin American region is immersed in the mental health concept. This is also part of the generic notion of public health and therefore involves the pragmatic application of knowledge in various fields: clinical, epidemiological, neurobiological, sociocultural, and basic research, as the most important ones. The objective is the normal development of individuals and the maintenance of integrally emotional functions at individual and collective level (Ustun and Sartorius 1995).

Mental health in the region has its origin in the establishment of specific programs within the regional office of WHO, the Pan American Health Organization (PAHO) in Washington, D.C. PAHO convened in 1962, the first mental health seminar in the Latin American region in Mexico City (PAHO 1980).

The Declaration of Caracas in 1990 (González and Levav 1990) reiterated that conventional psychiatric attention was not compatible with a necessary assistance based on the principles of community intervention, decentralization, participation, integration, and preventive measures in addition to treatment and rehabilitation. Specific suggestions were made in relation to the development of national mental health programs in Latin countries, community campaigns, control of affective disorders, epilepsy and psychosis, promoting mental health and psychosocial development of children, increase of vocational training centers, and improved legislation and regulations for the protection of human rights (Brody 1985).

In 2008, PAHO approved the 2008–2012 Strategic Plan with one among other objectives to prevent and reduce the burden of disease, disability, and premature death related to noncommunicable diseases, mental disorders, violence, and injuries. On the other hand, the Health Agenda for the Americas 2008 proposes eight priority areas: strengthening the authority of national health agencies, examining the socioeconomic determinants of health, enhancing social protection and access to services, decreasing the inequalities in health care within countries and between countries in

S. D. Monsalve (✉)
Department of Psychosomatic Medicine and Psychotherapy,
University Medical Center, Hauptstr. 8, 79104 Freiburg, Germany
e-mail: sonia.diaz-monsalve@uniklinik-freiburg.de

K. Fritzsche et al. (eds.), *Psychosomatic Medicine,* DOI 10.1007/978-1-4614-1022-5_18,

the region, reducing the risks and burden of diseases, developing the workforce in the health sector, and utilizing properly the knowledge of science and technology, all within a high bioethical context (PAHO 2009).

Mari et al. (2009) described that there are phases in the process of research on psychiatric epidemiology in Latin America. The first phase included the study of "Psychosomatic maladjustment syndrome" described in Andean migrants living in marginal areas of Lima, Peru (Seguín 1951). The second phase started with the development of standardized instruments, screening interviews, and questionnaires properly validated, following American US models. The data of all epidemiological studies are collected by the database Latin American and Caribbean Health Sciences (LILACS) between 1999 and 2008 focused on issues such as domestic violence, depression or alcohol and substance abuse, tobacco, and drugs. The general prevalence of mental illness varied between 18 and 36 %. The specific rates for depression were 9–27 %, for alcohol abuse 7–57 %, for drug abuse 9–19 %.

Regarding mental health interventions, the "delayed treatment" is a phenomenon practically applicable to all Latin American countries in which some attention has been paid to patients with mental disorders. The burden of disease is very high considering its economic costs and the disability associated with both the individual and the family.

Regarding policy and mental health services, at present, 65 % of the countries in the region have specific mental health policy, 82 % have mental action plans, and 70 % have a specific legislation in this area. Approaches to mental health interventions have minor variations from country to country. Key principles are related to decentralization of services, inter-sectorial collaboration, multidisciplinary participation, and community support in treatment and rehabilitation. The slow translation of policy into service delivery in the region is shown in the following statistics: There are on average 5.4 psychiatric beds per 10,000 population, of which 4.6 (82.8 %) are in psychiatric hospitals and only 0.4 per 10,000 population in general hospitals (Alarcón 2002).

Regarding the work force in mental health services: The WHO Atlas on Mental Health (2005) shows for the Latin American and the Caribbean region a shortage of mental health professionals and a heterogeneous distribution within and among countries. The number of psychiatrists, for example, showed an average of 4.3 per 100,000 inhabitants; the extremes were 24 and 22.9 in Venezuela and Uruguay respectively, to 0.2 and 0.5 per 100,000 population in Guyana and El Salvador, respectively. Argentina had 106 psychologists per 100,000 inhabitants while Belize had none and Suriname and Trinidad Tobago only 0.2 and 0.3, respectively with a regional average of 10.3 per 100,000 population. The average does not reflect the large differences within and among countries.

It could be concluded that although there are still disparities, concrete actions have been implemented in the region to remove inequities. Some good examples are the training for mental primary health workers in Cali, Colombia; community psychiatry for marginalized urban areas in Tegucigalpa, Honduras and Porto Alegre, Brazil; community-university–state government collaboration in Mérida, Venezuela; extension of mental services in Santos, Brazil, support networks and social services in Medellin, Colombia; policy implementation in Black River, Argentina and care of victims of domestic violence in Monterrey, Mexico; community stress prevention clinics in Havana, Cuba; priority attention for patients with depression in Chile and prevention of addictions in La Paz, Bolivia (Alarcón 2002).

The challenge ahead in many countries of the region is to pay more attention to mental health by policy makers. The strategy of incorporating mental care in the field of primary care can be effective to a point but there is always the risk of placing mental health as subordinate of physical, when in reality research has clearly shown the opposite (Ustun and Sartorius 1995).

References

Alarcón RD. Salud Mental en América Latina: Circa 2002. In: Sepúlveda J, Editor. Salud panamericana en el siglo XXI. Fortalecimiento de la cooperación internacional y desarrollo de capital humano. México, D.F.: Instituto Nacional de Salud Pública; 2002.

Brody EB. Patient rights, a cultural challenge to Western psychiatry. Am J Psychiatry. 1985;194: 58–62.

González R, Levav I. Reestructuración de la atención psiquiátrica: Bases conceptuales y guías para su implementación. Memorias de la Conferencia Regional para la restructuración de la Atención Psiquiátrica. Caracas, Venezuela. Nov. 11–14, 1990. Washington, D.C.: Instituto Mario Negri Italia.

Mari JJ, García de Olveira B, Silva de Lima M, Levav I. Breve historia de la epidemiología psiquiátrica en América Latina y el Caribe. In: Rodríguez JJ, Kohn R, Aguilar S, Editors. Epidemiología de los trastornos mentales en América Latina y el Caribe. Washington, D.C.: Organización Panamericana de la Salud; 2009.

Organización Panamericana de la Salud Salud para todos en el año 2000. Estrategias. Washington, D.C.: Documento Oficial No. 173; 1980.

Roses M. Welcoming remarks to the regional advisory Committee on health Statistics (CRAES). August 11, Washington, D.C.: PAHO; 2009.

Seguín CA. Síndrome psicosomático de desadaptación. Rev Lat Am Psiquiatría. 1951;1:16–26.

Ustun T, Sartorius N. Mental health in general health care. Chichester: Wiley; 1995.

World Health Organization. Mental Health Atlas 2005 (Revised Edition). http://www.who.int/mental_health/evidence/mhatlas05/en/.

Chapter 19
Psychosomatic Medicine in Iran

Hamid Afshar Zanjani and Farzad Goli

Various mind–body control methods such as yoga, meditation, reiki, hypnosis, and music therapy could be mentioned as precursors of Psychosomatic Medicine in Iran.

Although psychosomatic practice has been considered in different settings and departments but the academic contacts with Psychosomatic Medicine departments traced back to the twenty-first century to the Iranian Journal of Higher Health (the first journal by biopsychosocial approach to medicine in Iran) and international congresses of 2008.

For development of Psychosomatic Medicine in Iran with a plenty of German faculties such as Freiburg and Ulm, and also Mental Health and Globalization in Iran, which was a 3-year (2009-2013) TOT program for health care professionals in coordination with psychosomatic department of Freiburg University, Isfahan University of Medical Sciences, and Danesh-e-Tandorosti Institute.

At the moment, there is a subspecialty program for psychiatrists at Tehran University of Medical Sciences. There are few numbers of psychosomatic clinics in Isfahan and Tehran and also one psychosomatic research center in Isfahan. Fortunately, there is a very powerful trend to psychosomatic health care services both in professional and popular health sectors, so an emergent development in these services would be anticipated. Several academic researches have been done in the field in recent years and there is an ever-rising number of physicians interested in Psychosomatic Medicine.

H. Afshar Zanjani (✉)
Department of Psychiatry, Medical Faculty, Psychosomatic Research Center,
Isfahan University of Medical Sciences, Isfahan, Iran
e-mail: afshar@med.mui.ac.ir, shafsharz@gmail.com

Noor Hospital, Isfahan, Iran

F. Goli
Department of bioenergy economy,
Energy Medicine University, California, USA
e-mail: Dr.fgoli@yahoo.com

Danesh-e Tandorosti Institute, Isfahan, Iran
e-mail: info@iranianhealth.com

K. Fritzsche et al. (eds.), *Psychosomatic Medicine,* DOI 10.1007/978-1-4614-1022-5_19,

Although Psychosomatic Medicine has had ancient roots in Iran since middle ages, the modern aspects in Iran is still young and need more time to be integrated into the health delivery system and also academic programs. To establish psychologists and psychiatrists who practice hypnotherapy, relaxation, mindfulness trainings, biofeedback, and psychotherapeutic interventions, we need an integrative set of epidemiological and cultural studies for adjusting the globalized knowledge and technology by the local demands and resources and designing optimized psychosomatic clinical settings and institutions.

Index

K. Fritzsche et al. (eds.), *Psychosomatic Medicine,* DOI 10.1007/978-1-4614-1022-5,

Printed by Printforce, the Netherlands